# Healthy *Snacks* for *Snack Lovers*

Zain Naqvi

Order this book online at www.trafford.com
or email orders@trafford.com

Most Trafford titles are also available at major online book retailers.

Print information available on the last page.

ISBN: 978-1-4907-5738-4 (sc)
ISBN: 978-1-4907-5737-7 (e)

*Trafford rev.  03/19/2015*

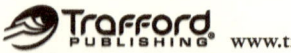 www.trafford.com

North America & international
toll-free: 1 888 232 4444 (USA & Canada)
fax: 812 355 4082

# Introduction

I love snacks. Be it chips, cookies, cakes, popcorn, I enjoy my fair share of them. Some common misconceptions about eating healthy are that you have to have a lot of time and a lot of money. That's absolutely not true. All eating healthy requires is for you to pay attention and take that extra step of looking at the nutrition label and the ingredients of your item and asking yourself if you think that the product is right to put in your body. In this book what I hope to do is made eating healthy a little easier. First of all I have presented an alternative to the nutrition label that you will find easier to read. Then I take all the snack foods that you love and evaluate if they are healthy, whether there is too much sugar or salt or high fructose corn syrup. If your favorite munchies aren't too good for you, I have provided a list of some healthy alternatives. Enjoy and hopefully pick up some healthy eating tips on the way. In this book I examine the following categories of snacks: Cookies, granola bar, crackers and chips.

## Glossary

## BASIC KNOWLEDGE:

**Before we get started I think it will help to understand some basic terms related to diet.**

## What is a calorie?

**Calories:** A calorie is the amount of energy that it takes to heat 1 gram of water to 1 degree Celsius. There are 4.18 joules in a calorie.

A simpler way to think about what a calorie actually is that a calorie is just a unit of energy or work. Work and energy are interchangeable concepts in Physics. So a calorie gives us a certain amount of energy that allows us to do a certain amount of work. Our energy comes from foods and therefore this is one way to look at different types of foods. For example if a food has 50 calories you can think that you are getting 50 units of energy from eating this food. Now too many calories are bad for you because if your body does not burn the calories, it stores them for leaner times. That storage is the excess fat in your body and stores that are too large are bad for your body for many reasons.

## What is fat?

Fat: Fat is a nutrient. It is crucial for normal body function and without it we could not live. Not only does fat supply us with energy, it also makes it possible for other nutrients to do their jobs. Some fats are liquid at room temperature while others are solid. We refer to those which are liquid at room temperature as *oils*. Eating too much fat is not good for you but they are healthy in moderation just like anything else.

Why do we need fats: storage of energy; cushion for organs; taste great. For the most part, starvation, rather than obesity, has been the main problem for our ancestors. Thus the fact that we find fat food tasty actually gave humans a survival advantage back when we had to hunt for food daily. Think of this as our very own refrigerator for lean times.

Saturated fats:

Fats are molecules which contain mostly carbon and hydrogen. The fats which have the maximum number of hydrogens (two hydrogens per carbon atom) are called **saturated**. As you can see below, each carbon is attached to two or more hydrogen atoms. This is a very compact structure and is therefore solid at room temperature. Saturated fat is an unhealthy fat that is naturally found in foods from animals such as fatty cuts of meat, poultry with the skin on and higher fat milk, cheese and yogurt. Saturated fat is also found in tropical oils, including coconut and palm oil.

Saturated Fat

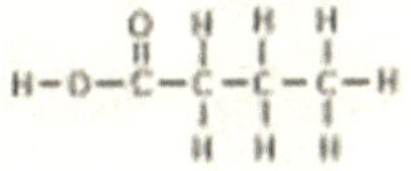

Monounsaturated Fat

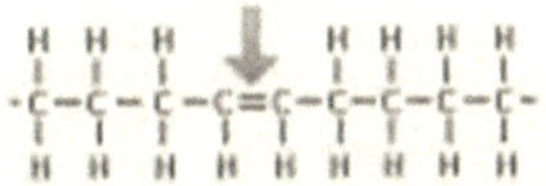

Polyunsaturated Fat

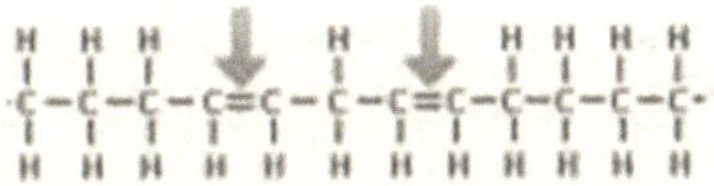

Unsaturated Fat: Unsaturated fat is a molecule which does not have the maximum number of hydrogen atoms attached to each carbon. These can then be called mono or polyunsaturated fats depending on how many hydrogens are missing. These tend to be less compact and are liquid at room temperature.

- **monounsaturated fat**, which can be found in foods like avocados, nuts and seeds

- **polyunsaturated fat**, which can be found in some types of fish, nuts seedoils.

We can take these healthy unsaturated fats and cook them with hydrogen and make **Trans fats.** Trans refers to a shape of the molecule. This process makes the fats more compact and thus can be solid at room temperature. While there are a few naturally occurring trans fats, most of the trans fats are man made. Trans fats are the unhealthiest fats that you should try to eat as little as possible of. These are commonly found in prepackaged foods such as breads, cakes, and pastries or fast food such as fries. We should try to eat as little of these foods as possible.

## *"Hydrogenated Oils"*

Oils have been hydrogenated for many decades, to prolong their shelf life and make the oils more stable. Hydrogenated oil is oil in which the essential fatty acids have been converted to a different form chemically, which has several effects. Hydrogenated oil is far more shelf stable, and will not go rancid as quickly as untreated oil. All medical professionals agree that people should limit their consumption of hydrogenated oil to avoid exposure to trans fats, and should eat foods with healthy fats such as nuts, avocados, and olive oil.

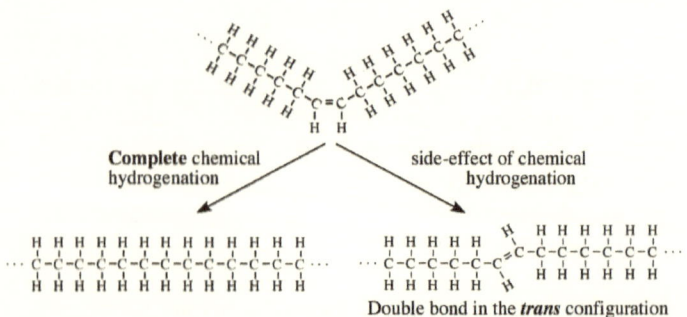

Complete chemical hydrogenation

side-effect of chemical hydrogenation

Double bond in the *trans* configuration

Thus in summary, there are saturated fats which are naturally occurring. There are unsaturated fats which are good and naturally occurring. Then there are trans fats which are mostly man made and are the worst for us. These are made by hydrogenating otherwise good fats so that they may be more solid.

Trans fats increase the level of cholesterol in the blood. Substituting saturated and trans fats with unsaturated fats has been shown to help lower cholesterol levels and reduce the risk of heart disease.

Cholesterol: Burgers. Cheese. Fries. What do all these foods have in common other than being delicious? They are all high in cholesterol. The first thing to understand about cholesterol is that when we talk about fat, we are generally talking about triglycerides, not cholesterol. Cholesterol, while it is waxy, fatty substance, is not the same as fat. It is a chemical which is needed by the body for cell membranes, hormones and some vitamins.

Our body produces 1000 mg of cholesterol a day so you would be perfectly fine if you didn't eat foods with any cholesterol in them. Nowadays it is hard to avid cholesterol because it is so common in foods. It helps to keep in mind that cholesterol is exclusively an animal product, not found in plants. Meats, egg yolks, butter, cheese all contain cholesterol. It is best to have as little cholesterol as possible. The reason for this is that excess cholesterol causes the blood vessels in our heart to block up and if the blockage is severe it can lead to a heart attack.

This is not to say that all cholesterol is bad. Our body packages two types of cholesterol; the Low density particles and High density particles. Low density cholesterol is bad and the High density cholesterol is good. A good way to remember is L for Lousy and we want it Lower and H for Happy and we want it Higher.

**Carbohydrates**: this is one of the most important parts of a food label. Why? Because this is where we can find out how much sugar is in our muffin or how much fiber is in our bagel.

Carbohydrates very simply come from Carbon and Hydrates. So the formula of carbohydrates is $C$ $H_2O$. The simplest carbohydrate has six carbons, twelve hydrogens and six oxygens. One such molecule is called a SACCHARIDE.

Simple sugars have one or two saccahrides. Complex carbohydrates have more than two saccharides.

The basic saccharides are glucose, fructose and galactose. Table sugar has glucose and fructose and is called sucrose. These simple sugars are easily broken down in the gut and get into the blood stream.

When many chains of these sugars are made, they form chains that can be easily broken down in the gut called starches. These thus quickly become multiple molecules of simple sugars in the gut and raise blood sugar levels.

Other chains of sugars are made in such a way that they cannot be broken down in the gut and these are called fiber and therefore do not raise blood sugar levels. Fiber is either insoluble or soluble. Soluble fiber is that which breaks down with water eg. oatmeal. Insoluble does not break down with water eg broccoli. As fiber goes through our body, it drags with it some toxins, reduces absorption of some simple carbohydrates, and keeps the gut moving. means that our body does not digest it. Instead it goes right through our digestive tract and come out in our stool. It is very good for us as it helps our digestion and helps our body excrete waste.

Carbohydrates are used as the main source of energy for the body. If there are excessive amounts of carbohydrates ingested, then these are stored as glycogen. Further amounts are converted into triglycerides or fat. This, in turn lead to obesity, metabolic syndrome and Type 2 diabetes. So, for instance, high fructose corn syrup, which is high in simple carbohydrates is felt to be the real driver of the current epidemic of Type 2 diabetes, heart attacks, strokes, cancer, and possibly even dementia.

When you add the amount of sugar, starch and fiber you get the total amount of carbohydrates in the food. On most labels, you will find the total amount of carbohydrates and sugars but they often only give you the fiber and not the starches. **Subtracting the fiber from the total carbohydrates thus gives you the "bad carbs" of that food.**

**Protein**: The last part of the food label is protein. Protein is an essential nutrient for our body. So essential is protein to our body that the word comes from the Greek word "protos" or first. So it is the first type of food, necessary for growth, maintenance, enzyme activity and most essential body functions. Our bodies like foods with high protein also because they are a great fuel and get converted easily to energy.

Proteins are made up of chains of molecules called amino acids. There are in all twenty amino acids which can be thought of as letters of the alphabet. Arranged in different sequences, these amino acids will lead to different proteins much as the alphabet can be arranged in many ways to give different words. Rather than to think of the twenty amino acids, it is easier to think of essential and non-essential amino acids. Essential are those which our body cannot make and non-essential are those which our body can make. Thus we must get essential amino acids in our diet.

Foods which contain all the essential amino acids are considered to be complete source of protein. These include mostly animal products and only one plant product (soy bean). The way vegetarians get full complement of essential amino acids is by combining grain and lentils for instance. The essential amino acid missing in lentils can be found in grains. This explains the historic practice of lentils and rice/ bread in India and beans and tacos in South America.

People often worry too much about having excess amounts of protein. Unless the person has kidney disease this is actually hard to do.

### *"Salt/Sodium"*

This is a pretty obvious and well known fact that too much salt is bad for you. You can say whether or not there is a lot of salt in a food because the higher the ingredient is on the list the more of it is in the food. Too much salt can lead to high blood pressure, stroke, and possibly stomach cancer.

# How to read a nutrition label

This page maybe the most important part of the book. In fact if you just read this page and nothing else, I think buying this book would have been worthwhile (which is not to say that you shouldn't read the book!). The reason for this is that on this page, I am going to teach you a life skill. The skill is called "how to read a nutrition label and a ingredient list". Nowadays every food item that comes in a package must come with a nutrition label and an ingredient list. This allows us to know exactly what we are putting into our bodies and helps us make good food choices. Reading a nutrition label is an extremely important skill to have so that we can always be able to make healthy food choices even when the food comes pre packaged. An ingredient list is also essential because you want to know what you are putting in your body when you are eating a pre packaged food

So let us look at this in detail. You will find generally on food labels two sections. The first one is the "Nutrition facts" section.

# Nutrition Facts

Serving Size 1/2 cup dry (40 g)
Servings Per container: 13

Amount Per Serving

**Calories** 150          Calories from Fat 25

| | % Daily Value* |
|---|---|
| **Total Fat** 3 g | 4% |
| Saturated Fat 0.5 g | 2% |
| Trans Fat 0 g | 0% |
| **Cholesterol** 0 mg | 0% |
| **Sodium** 0 mg | 0% |
| **Total Carbohydrate** 27 g | 9% |
| Dietary Fiber 4 g | 15% |
| Sugars 1 g | |
| **Protein** 5 g | |
| Vitamin A | 0% |
| Vitamin C | 0% |
| Calcium | 0% |
| Iron | 10% |

*Percent Daily Values are based on a 2,000 calorie diet.
Your daily values may be higher or lower depending on
your calorie needs.

The second is the list of ingredients and you must see both.

Lets start with the Nutrition Facts.

The first thing to note is the serving size. This is important to note so that when you are comparing two products for example, you need to make sure you are comparing nutrients for the same serving size e.g ½ cup on both products.

The next section is total fat. This, you will recall is made up of saturated, unsaturated and trans fats. The only good fat is the unsaturated fats. So in the example we have, the 3 grams represent total fats. 0.5g is saturated and there is no trans fats. Thus it has 2.5g unsaturated fats. Here, it is important to note that if the food contains 0.5g trans fats, they can get away with not mentioning it. The way to check this is to look in the list of ingredients. If it has "hydrogenated" or partially hydrogenated oils, then it has trans fats.

The next section is carbohydrates. Total carbohydrates is fiber + sugars + starch. The good carbohydrate is fiber. Best way to sort out how much sugar or starch is present is to subtract fiber from the total carbohydrates. In our label, there are 27g of carbohydrates and 4g of fiber. Thus this product has 23g of sugar or starch (bad carbs). If you wish to confirm that the food is high in fiber, look on the ingredients list. It should have the word "whole" before the grain e.g wheat, oats or rye.

Sodium is an important ingredient to look at. Daily intake of sodium should be about 2g or preferably 1500mg.

Most of the ingredianets that I cannot pronounce make me want to reject that item as a food choice. The ones to watch out for in particular include nitrites and nitrates, which could interact with medications to damage DNA and increase the risk of cancer.

I generally avoid looking at the segments on vitamins etc. I do not pay much attention to the % daily intake section as well. Our body has different requirements at different stages of life. So how can the percentage daily intake for a growing body be the same as for someone who is old. Also our nutritional requirements depend on our activity, lifestyle etc. So a marathon runner would require more than a sedentary individual. I find this very misleading and am surprised more people have not been led astray as a result.

The next big section to look at is the ingredient list, which shows all the ingredients in a packaged food.
Ingredients are listed in order of weight, beginning with the ingredient that weighs the most and ending

with the ingredient that weighs the least. This means that a food contains *more* of the ingredients found at the beginning of the list, and *less* of the ingredients at the end of the list. For example if sugar is the first ingredient in the list, it is probably something that you should avoid because there is a lot of sugar in the product in proportion to anything else. However, things are not that simple. For instance sugar can be hidden in many forms including corn syrup, agave nectar, barley malt syrup or another chemical ending in –ose.

***Look also for chemicals and words you cannot pronounce. If they are high on the list, avoid that product.***

Here are another couple of things you should be aware of in the list of ingredients.

### *"Corn Syrup"*

High fructose corn syrup (HFCS)— which can have many names depending on the country including glucose-fructose or Isoglucose contains a syrup which has had some glucose chemically converted to fructose (to make it sweeter). Because of its low price, HFCS is the commonest sweetener used in processed foods and beverages in the United States. The chemical process makes the fructose and glucose readily absorbed and liver turns the excess into fats.

### Monosodium glutamate

MSG is often added to foods to preserve them and also to make them taste better. It does this by tricking your tongue, using a little-known fifth basic taste: umami.

Umami is the taste of glutamate, which is a savory flavor found in many Japanese foods and bacon. Foods containing MSG taste heartier, more robust and generally better to a lot of people than foods without it.

One of the best overviews of the very real dangers of MSG comes from Dr. Russell Blaylock, a board-certified neurosurgeon and author of *"Excitotoxins: The Taste that Kills."* In it he explains that MSG is an excitotoxin, which means it overexcites your cells to the point of damage or death, causing brain damage to varying degrees—and potentially even triggering or worsening learning disabilities, Alzheimer's disease, Parkinson's disease, Lou Gehrig's disease and more.

While some other studies have not shown such risk, I think foods containing MSG should probably be avoided as some people can get a reaction to the MSG. This causes headache, flushing, sweating, fluttering heartbeat, and shortness of breath.

We will get more practice at this as we go through the book.

## Other Tricks To Watch Out For:

### *"Low Fat/Reduced Fat"*

Nutrient claims such as 'low fat' are often used by food manufacturers to point out the nutrition benefits of their product.

Manufacturers who use this claim have to make sure the product meets strict criteria before they are allowed to print 'low in fat' on the food label.

A 'low fat' or 'low in fat' food must contain no more than 3g of fat per 100g of food. A liquid must contain no more than 1.5g fat per 100g.

'Reduced fat' means the food must contain at least 25% less fat than the regular product to which it is being compared, and at least 3g less fat per 100g of food.

This means that a product can still be relatively high in fat, but still labeled reduced fat. And as a side note, most products that have low fat or reduced fat make up for the lack of fat with an increase in the sugar so there is no real benefit.

## PRACTISING THE SKILL

So lets look at the ingredients of a packaged product which happens to be one of the most popular snacks in the world: an oreo cookie.

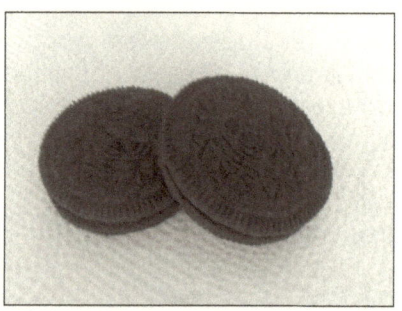

SUGAR, UNBLEACHED ENRICHED FLOUR (WHEAT FLOUR, NIACIN, REDUCED IRON, THIAMINE MONONITRATE {VITAMIN B1}, RIBOFLAVIN {VITAMIN B2}, FOLIC ACID), HIGH OLEIC CANOLA AND/OR PALM AND/OR CANOLA AND/OR SOYBEAN OIL, COCOA (PROCESSED WITH ALKALI), HIGH FRUCTOSE CORN SYRUP, CORNSTARCH, LEAVENING (BAKING SODA AND/OR CALCIUM PHOSPHATE), SALT, SOY LECITHIN, VANILLIN—AN ARTIFICIAL FLAVOR,

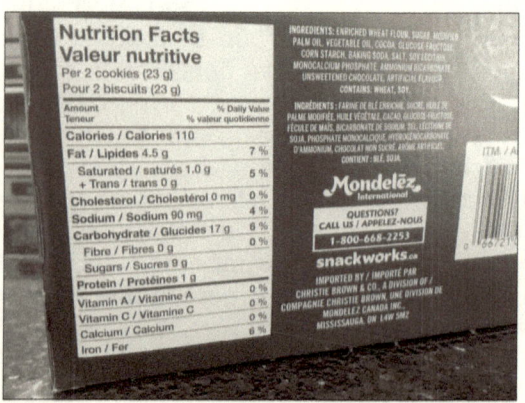

We can see that sadly the very first ingredient is Enriched wheat flour, This means that the ingredient there is most of in an oreo is wheat flour. The second ingredient is sugar. This means that the second largest amount of one ingredient in the cookie is sugar. Next up is oil although they do not specify which one it has (this we will sort out in the nutrition facts). It also has corn syrup and cornstarch. So okay we already know that corn syrup is bad but what is corn starch? Well corn starch is a thickening agent that has starch. It is thus very sugary but has no vitamins or minerals and so it is just best that it should be eaten in moderation if at all.

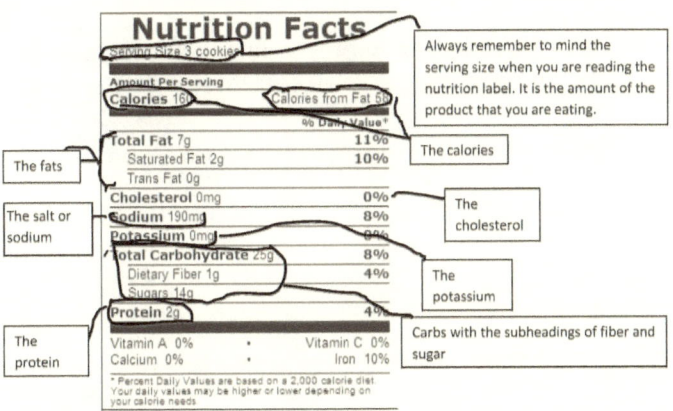

Actually if you look near the top of the label, you will see that the serving size of this nutrition label is not 1 but **2 cookies**.

Then if you look under the serving size you will see that the calories for two oreos are 110 calories or around 53 per cookie. A little of the left of the calories you will see that 60 of these 160 calories are from fat! The rest are probably carbohydrates but let's read on.

On the NUTRITION FACTS section I pay attention to the GRAMS. So two cookies weigh 23 g. Of these 4.5 g are fat, 17g are carbohydrates and 1g are protein.

Of the 4.5 g of fats, 1g are saturated fats and transfat. The rest are unsaturated fats.

Of the 17 g of carbohydrates, 1g is fiber the rest is either sugar or starch, which is all bad for us.

## SO IN SUMMERY:
## POSTITIVES

- Convenient
- Portable
- Cheap
- Tasty
- Some effort has been made to use unsaturated fats that are better than saturated and trans fat.

## NEGETIVES

- High bad carbs content (including HFCS)
- High fat content
- High calorie
- Low protein and fiber

## The verdict

Though very tasty and convenient, it is not a healthy snack by any means because of the high fat and sugar content as well as the low nutritional profile. Oreos should only be eaten sparingly as a treat not an everyday snack.

Hopefully this has given you some confidence in reading labels. Now we will look at different food categories to find out the healthiest option in each category.

# MY Proposed Rating Scale -10 Stars System

Understanding food labels and going through the ingredient list is time consuming. I have therefore made a simple rating scale, which is basically 10 Stars. This allows people to read label quicker. The explanation for the stars is as follows:

10 Star criteria for evaluating snacks.

First we assign 10 stars to all the products and then we go through the ingredient list and deduct points for the following.

**Carbohyrates**

| | | |
|---|---|---|
| Total carbs minus fiber | > 30% by weight | -1 |
| Total carbs minus fiber | > 50% by weight | -2 |
| Fiber | < 5% by weight | -1 |
| **Fats** | | |
| Fat | > 20 % by weight | -1 |
| Saturated / Trans fats | | -1 |
| **Proteins** | < 10% by weight | -1 |
| Sodium | > 1 mg/ calories | -1 |
| Cholesterol | > 1mg /20 calories | -1 |
| Minerals and Vitamins absent | | -1 |
| Additives | | -1 |

Therefore maximum is 10 stars and minimum is 0.

# Cookie

Cookies appear to have their origins in 7th century AD <u>Persia</u>, not too long after the practice of using sugar became relatively common in the region.[1] Cookies made their way to Europe through the <u>Muslim conquest of Spain</u>. By the 14th century, cookies were common in all ranks of society throughout Europe, from royal cuisine to street vendors.

With global travel becoming widespread at that time, cookies made a great travel companion, a modernized equivalent of the travel cakes used throughout history. One of the most popular early cookies, which traveled especially well and became known on every continent by similar names, was the **<u>Jumble</u>**, a relatively hard cookie mostly made of nuts, sweetener, and water.

Cookies arrived in America after the early English settlement (the 17th century), although the name "koekje" arrived with the Dutch. This became Anglicized to "cookie" or **cooky**. The popular early American cookies were the <u>macaroon</u>, <u>gingerbread cookies</u>, and of course jumbles of various types.

The most common modern cookie, styled by the cream made of butter and sugar, was not common until the 18th century. As delectable as they are, cookies, sadly are unhealthy. They tend to have high fats and sugar without any additional nutritional content. I would not really recommend having cookies as a snack every day because of the amount of sugars and fats. However, once in a while they are fine. Just a heads up most of the products on this list cookie will get a bad rating because they are after all cookies.

# Nabisco Oreo Double Stuff Chocolate Sandwich Cookie

## Nutrition Facts

Serving Size 3 cookies

**Amount Per Serving**

| Calories 160 | Calories from Fat 58 |
|---|---|

| | % Daily Value* |
|---|---|
| **Total Fat** 7g | 11% |
| Saturated Fat 2g | 10% |
| Trans Fat 0g | |
| **Cholesterol** 0mg | 0% |
| **Sodium** 190mg | 8% |
| **Potassium** 0mg | 0% |
| **Total Carbohydrate** 25g | 8% |
| Dietary Fiber 1g | 4% |
| Sugars 14g | |
| **Protein** 2g | 4% |

| Vitamin A 0% | • | Vitamin C 0% |
|---|---|---|
| Calcium 0% | • | Iron 10% |

* Percent Daily Values are based on a 2,000 calorie diet. Your daily values may be higher or lower depending on your calorie needs.

**Ingredients**: SUGAR, UNBLEACHED ENRICHED FLOUR (WHEAT FLOUR, NIACIN, REDUCED IRON, THIAMINE MONONITRATE {VITAMIN B1}, RIBOFLAVIN {VITAMIN B2}, FOLIC ACID), HIGH OLEIC CANOLA AND/OR PALM AND/OR CANOLA OIL, COCOA (PROCESSED WITH ALKALI), HIGH FRUCTOSE CORN SYRUP, CORNSTARCH, LEAVENING (BAKING SODA AND/OR CALCIUM PHOSPHATE), SALT, SOY LECITHIN, VANILLIN—AN ARTIFICIAL FLAVOR, CHOCOLATE.

No cholesterol, High fat, High sugar, Low protein, Lots of sugar, corn starch, corn syrup, salt

**Rating**: 2.5/10 stars

# Chips Ahoy Original

## NUTRITION FACTS

Serving Size: 40 g
Serving per container about 12

**Amount Per Serving**

Calories 190

Calories from Fat 80

| | % Daily Value* |
|---|---|
| Total Fat 9g | 14% |
| Saturated Fat 3g | 15% |
| Trans Fat 0g | 0% |
| Monounsaturated Fat 2g | 0% |
| Cholesterol 0mg | 0% |
| Sodium 120mg | 5% |
| Potassium 50mg | 1% |
| Total Carbohydrate 27g | 9% |
| Dietary Fiber 1g | 4% |
| Sugars 13g | |
| Protein 2g | |

| Vitamin A 0% | Calcium 0% |
|---|---|
| Vitamin C 0% | Iron 6% |

*Percent Daily Values are based on a 2,000 calorie diet. Your daily values may be higher or lower depending on your calorie needs:

| | Calories: | 2,000 | 2,500 |
|---|---|---|---|
| Total Fat | Less than | 65g | 80g |
| Sat Fat | Less than | 20g | 25g |
| Cholest | Less than | 300mg | 300mg |
| Sodium | Less than | 2,400mg | 2,400mg |
| Total Carb | | 300g | 375g |
| Fiber | | 25g | 30g |

**INGREDIENTS**: UNBLEACHED ENRICHED FLOUR (WHEAT FLOUR, NIACIN, REDUCED IRON, THIAMINE MONONITRATE {VITAMIN B1}, RIBOFLAVIN {VITAMIN B2}, FOLIC ACID), SEMISWEET CHOCOLATE CHIPS (SUGAR, CHOCOLATE, COCOA BUTTER, DEXTROSE, SOY LECITHIN), SUGAR, SOYBEAN OIL AND/OR PARTIALLY HYDROGENATED COTTONSEED OIL, HIGH FRUCTOSE CORN SYRUP, LEAVENING (BAKING SODA AND/OR AMMONIUM PHOSPHATE), SALT, WHEY (FROM MILK), NATURAL AND ARTIFICIAL FLAVOR, CARAMEL COLOR. CONTAINS: WHEAT, SOY, MILK

Contains high fructose corn syrup, salt, very few "real" ingredients, has 0 cholesterol, high salt, fat, sugar, Low protein, fiber, high calorie
**Rating**: 3/10 stars

# The Decadent

| Nutrition Facts / Valeur nutritive | |
|---|---|
| Per 2 cookies (34 g) / pour 2 biscuits (34 g) | |
| **Amount / Teneur** | **% Daily Value / % valeur quotidienne** |
| **Calories / Calories** 170 | |
| **Fat / Lipides** 8 g | 12 % |
| Saturates / saturés 5 g + Trans / trans 0.1 g | 26 % |
| **Cholesterol / Cholestérol** 25 mg | |
| **Sodium / Sodium** 85 mg | 4 % |
| **Carbohydrate / Glucides** 23 g | 8 % |
| Fibre / Fibres 1 g | 4 % |
| Sugars / Sucres 13 g | |
| **Protein / Protéines** 2 g | |
| Vitamin A / Vitamine A | 4 % |
| Vitamin C / Vitamine C | 0 % |
| Calcium / Calcium | 2 % |
| Iron / Fer | 10 % |

**Ingredients**: CHOCOLATE CHIPS (UNSWEETENED CHOCOLATE, SUGAR, DEXTEROSE, COCOA BUTTER, SOY LECITHIN, VANILLA EXTRACT), ENRICHED WHEAT FLOUR, BUTTER, BROWN SUGAR, SUGAR, COCONUT (CONTAINS SULOHITES), MODIFIED MILK INGREDINTS, DREID WHOLE EGGS, BAKING SODA, VANILLA EXTRACT, SALT. MAY CONTAIN PENUTS AND TREE NUTS.

Summary: High calorie, high fat, high cholesterol, high carbs, low protein, low fiber, real ingredients, relatively low sodium

Carbs -2
Fats -2
Low protein -1
Cholesterol -1
Low fibre -1
Nutrition -.5
**Rating**: 2.5/10 stars

# Pepperidge Farm:
## Double Chocolate Chunk Dark Chocolate

## Cookie

## Nutrition Facts

Serving Size 28 g
Servings Per Container 8

**Amount Per Serving**

| **Calories** 140 | Calories from Fat 60 |
|---|---|

| | % Daily Value* |
|---|---|
| **Total Fat** 7 g | **11%** |
| Saturated Fat 3 g | **15%** |
| Trans Fat 0 g | |
| **Cholesterol** 10 mg | **3%** |
| **Sodium** 80 mg | **3%** |
| **Total Carbohydrate** 18 g | **6%** |
| Dietary Fiber 1 g | **4%** |
| Sugars 10 g | |
| **Protein** 2 g | |

| Vitamin A | 0 |
|---|---|
| Vitamin C | 0 |
| Calcium | 0 |
| Iron | 6% |

Carbs -2
Fats -2
Low protein -1
Cholesterol -1
Low fibre -1
Nutrition -1
Rating: 2/10

Semi-Sweet Chocolate (Sugar, Chocolate Liquor, Cocoa Butter, Dextrose, Soy Lecithin Added As An Emulsifier, Vanilla Extract), Unbleached Enriched Wheat Flour [Flour, Niacin, Reduced Iron, Thiamin Mononitrate (Vitamin B1), Riboflavin (Vitamin B2), Folic Acid], Sugar, Vegetable Oils (Palm and/Or Interesterified and Hydrogenated Cottonseed), Butter (Milk), Whole Eggs, Brown Sugar, Contains 2 Percent Or Less of: Leavening (Baking Soda, Ammonium Bicarbonate, Cream of Tartar), Butter Oil, Salt, Natural Flavor and Caramel Color.

## Nabisco Oreo Double Stuff
## Golden Sandwich Cookies, 15.25 oz

# Nutrition Facts

Serving Size 30 G
Servings Per Container 14

**Amount Per Serving**

**Calories** 150          Calories from Fat 60

% **Daily Value\***

| | |
|---|---|
| **Total Fat** 7 G | **11** |
| Saturated Fat 2 G | **10** |
| Trans Fat 0 G | |
| Monounsaturated Fat 3.5 G | |
| **Cholesterol** 0 Mg | **0** |
| **Sodium** 80 Mg | **3** |
| **Potassium** 15 Mg | **0** |
| **Total Carbohydrate** 21 G | **7** |
| Dietary Fiber 0 G | **0** |
| Sugars 13 G | |
| **Protein** <1 G | |

| | |
|---|---|
| Vitamin A | 0 |
| Vitamin C | 0 |
| Calcium | 0 |

Carbs -2
Fats -2
Low protein -1
Low fiber -1
Nutrition -1
Preservatives -1

Rating 2/10

# Pepperidge Farm Soft Baked Cookies, Captiva Dark Chocolate Brownie, 8.6-ounce (pack of 5)

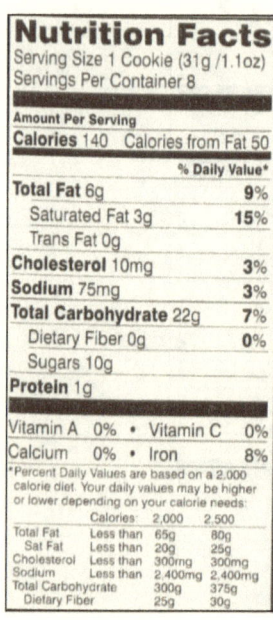

**Nutrition Facts**
Serving Size 1 Cookie (31g /1.1oz)
Servings Per Container 8

**Amount Per Serving**

**Calories** 140    Calories from Fat 50

| | % Daily Value* |
|---|---|
| **Total Fat** 6g | 9% |
| Saturated Fat 3g | 15% |
| Trans Fat 0g | |
| **Cholesterol** 10mg | 3% |
| **Sodium** 75mg | 3% |
| **Total Carbohydrate** 22g | 7% |
| Dietary Fiber 0g | 0% |
| Sugars 10g | |
| **Protein** 1g | |

| | | | |
|---|---|---|---|
| Vitamin A 0% | • | Vitamin C | 0% |
| Calcium 0% | • | Iron | 8% |

*Percent Daily Values are based on a 2,000 calorie diet. Your daily values may be higher or lower depending on your calorie needs:

| | Calories: | 2,000 | 2,500 |
|---|---|---|---|
| Total Fat | Less than | 65g | 80g |
| Sat Fat | Less than | 20g | 25g |
| Cholesterol | Less than | 300mg | 300mg |
| Sodium | Less than | 2,400mg | 2,400mg |
| Total Carbohydrate | | 300g | 375g |
| Dietary Fiber | | 25g | 30g |

**MADE FROM:** UNBLEACHED ENRICHED WHEAT FLOUR (FLOUR, NIACIN, REDUCED IRON, THIAMINE MONONITRATE [VITAMIN B1], RIBOFLAVIN [VITAMIN B2], FOLIC ACID), SEMI SWEET CHOCOLATE (SUGAR, CHOCOLATE LIQUOR, COCOA BUTTER, DEXTROSE, SOY LECITHIN, VANILLA EXTRACT), FRUCTOSE, SUGAR, BUTTER, VEGETABLE OILS (PALM AND/OR INTERESTERIFIED AND HYDROGENATED SOYBEAN AND/OR HYDROGENATED COTTONSEED), CORN SYRUP SOLIDS, COCOA PROCESSED WITH ALKALI (DUTCHED), CONTAINS 2 PERCENT OR LESS OF: CORNSTARCH, EGGS, NONFAT MILK, LEAVENING (BAKING SODA, CREAM OF TARTAR, AMMONIUM BICARBONATE), SALT AND NATURAL FLAVORS.

Carbs -2
Fats -1.5
Low protein -1
Cholesterol -1
Low fiber -1
Nutrition -1
Rating: 3/10 Stars

# FAMOUS AMOS

## Nutrition Facts

Serving Size 4 Cookies (29g)

**Amount Per Serving**

**Calories** 150    Calories from Fat 60

| | % Daily Value* |
|---|---|
| **Total Fat** 7g | **11%** |
| Saturated Fat 3g | **15%** |
| *Trans* Fat 0g | |
| **Cholesterol** less than 5mg | **1%** |
| **Sodium** 105mg | **4%** |
| **Total Carbohydrate** 20g | **7%** |
| Dietary Fiber less than 1g | **3%** |
| Sugars 9g | |
| **Protein** 1g | |

| | | | |
|---|---|---|---|
| Vitamin A | 0% | Vitamin C | 0% |
| Calcium | 0% | Iron | 2% |

* Percent Daily Values are based on a 2,000 calorie diet. Your daily values may be higher or lower depending on your calorie needs:

| | Calories | 2,000 | 2,500 |
|---|---|---|---|
| Total Fat | Less than | 65g | 80g |
| Sat. Fat | Less than | 20g | 25g |
| Cholesterol | Less than | 300mg | 300mg |
| Sodium | Less than | 2,400mg | 2,400mg |
| Total Carbohydrate | | 300g | 375g |
| Dietary Fiber | | 25g | 30g |

Calories per gram: Fat 9 • Carbohydrate 4 • Protein 4

**INGREDIENTS:** ENRICHED FLOUR (WHEAT FLOUR, NIACIN, REDUCED IRON, THIAMIN MONONITRATE [VITAMIN B₁], RIBOFLAVIN [VITAMIN B₂], FOLIC ACID), SEMISWEET CHOCOLATE (SUGAR, CHOCOLATE, COCOA BUTTER, SOY LECITHIN, NATURAL FLAVOR), SUGAR, VEGETABLE OIL (SOYBEAN, PALM, AND PALM KERNEL OIL WITH TBHQ FOR FRESHNESS). CONTAINS TWO PERCENT OR LESS OF MOLASSES, SALT, EGGS, BAKING SODA, NATURAL AND ARTIFICIAL FLAVOR, WHEY, WHEY PROTEIN CONCENTRATE.

**CONTAINS WHEAT, SOY, EGG AND MILK INGREDIENTS. MAY CONTAIN TREE NUTS.**

Carbs -2
Fats -2
Low protein -1
Cholesterol -1
Low fiber -1
Nutrition -1
Rating: 3/10

## Dads Cookies

# Nutrition Facts
Serving Size 2 each (35 g)

| Per Serving | % Daily Value* |
|---|---|
| **Calories** 170 | |
| Calories from Fat 54 | |
| **Total Fat** 6g | 9% |
| Saturated Fat 2g | 10% |
| **Cholesterol** 0mg | 0% |
| **Sodium** 180mg | 8% |
| **Carbohydrates** 28g | 9% |
| Dietary Fiber 1g | 4% |
| Sugars 13g | |
| **Protein** 2g | |

Vitamin A 0% · Vitamin C 0%

Calcium 0% · Iron 6%

- High calorie
- High fat
- LOTS OF SODIUM
- High carb, surprisingly low fiber for an oatmeal cookie
- Obviously tasty, portable

Rating: 2/10 stars

## Lil Debbie oat meal crème pies

**Nutrition Facts**
Serving Size 1 cookie (38 g)

| Per Serving | % Daily Value* |
|---|---|
| **Calories** 170 | |
| Calories from Fat 63 | |
| **Total Fat** 7g | 11% |
| Saturated Fat 2g | 10% |
| Polyunsaturated Fat 0g | |
| Monounsaturated Fat 0g | |
| **Cholesterol** 0mg | 0% |
| **Sodium** 170mg | 7% |
| **Potassium** 0mg | 0% |
| **Carbohydrates** 26g | 9% |
| Dietary Fiber 1g | 4% |
| Sugars 12g | |
| **Protein** 1g | |

Vitamin A 0% · Vitamin C 0%
Calcium 0% · Iron 4%

Corn Syrup, Enriched Bleached Flour (Wheat Flour, Barley Malt, Niacin, Reduced Iron, Thiamine Mononitrate [Vitamin B1], Riboflavin [Vitamin B2], Folic Acid), Vegetable Shortening (Partially Hydrogenated Soybean And Cottonseed Oils), Sugar, Oats, Water, Dextrose, Molasses, Raisins, Contains 2% Or Less Of Each Of The Following: Leavening (Baking Soda, Ammonium Bicarbonate), Whey (Milk), Salt, Emulsifiers (Soy Lecithin, Mono- And Diglycerides, Sorbitan Monostearate, Polysorbate 60), Corn Starch, Eggs, Egg Whites, Cocoa, Coconut (Sulfite Treated To Preserve Color), Evaporated Apples (Sulfite Treated To Preserve Color), Rice Flour, Nonfat Dry Milk, Carrageenan, Colors (Caramel Color, Yellow 5, Red 40), Sorbic Acid (To Retain Freshness), Spices, Natural And Artificial Flavors.

Negetives:
big
high fat, carb, low protein, fiber, high cals

Rating: 1.5 stars

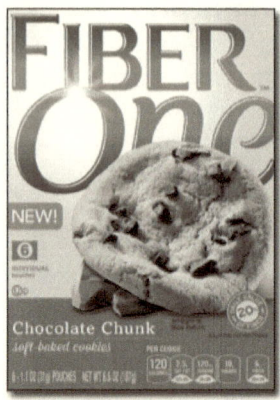
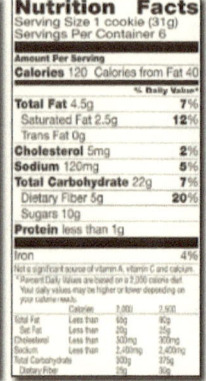
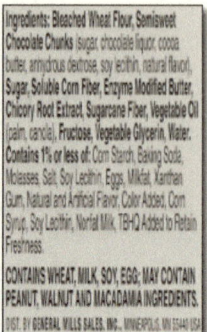

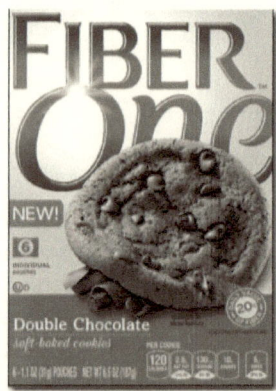
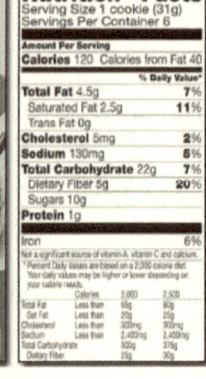

Lower then average calorie
Lower then average carbs
Lower then average fat
High fiber
High protein then average

Rating: 5/10 stars

## Nabisco Nilla Vanilla Wafers

### Nutrition Facts

Serving Size 8 wafers (33 g)

| Per Serving | % Daily Value* |
|---|---|
| Calories 140 | |
| Calories from Fat 54 | |
| Total Fat 6g | 9% |
| Saturated Fat 1.5g | 7% |
| Cholesterol 5mg | 2% |
| Sodium 115mg | 5% |
| Potassium 30mg | 1% |
| Carbohydrates 21g | 7% |
| Dietary Fiber 0g | 0% |
| Sugars 11g | |
| Protein 1g | |

Vitamin A 0% · Vitamin C 0%

Calcium 2% · Iron 4%

*Unbleached enriched flour (wheat flour, niacin, reduced iron, thiamine mononitrate {vitamin B1}, riboflavin {vitamin B2}, folic acid), sugar, soybean oil, high fructose corn syrup, partially hydrogenated cottonseed oil, whey (from milk), eggs, natural and artificial flavor, salt, leavening (baking soda and/or calcium phosphate), emulsifiers (mono- and diglycerides).* **Contains:** *Wheat, milk, egg, soy.*

I like these because they are small, portable, and so that makes it very easy to control your portions.

High fat, sodium, carb,

Rating: 4/10 Stars

# Pepridge farm Milano cookies

## Pepperidge Farm® Cookies

*Milano® Cookies*

**Nutrition Facts***
Amount per Serving (serving size) = 3 cookies

| | |
|---|---|
| Calories 180 | Sugars 11g |
| Fat Calories 80 | Protein 2g |
| Total Fat 9g | |
| Sat. Fat 4g | **% Daily Values**** |
| Trans Fat 0g | Vitamin A 0% |
| Cholesterol 5mg | Vitamin C 0% |
| Sodium 60mg | Calcium 0% |
| Total Carb. 22g | Iron 8% |
| Dietary Fiber 1g | |

* The nutrition information contained in this list of Nutrition Facts is based on our current data. However, because the data may change from time to time, this information may not always be identical to the nutritional label information of products on shelf.

** % Daily Values (DV) are based on a 2,000 calorie diet.

Wheat Flour Unbleached Enriched (Flour, Niacin Vitamin B3, Iron Reduced, Thiamine Mononitrate Vitamin B1[Thiamin Vitamin B1], Riboflavin Vitamin B2 [Riboflavin Vitamin B2], Folic Acid Vitamin B9), Sugar, Vegetables Oil (Palm Kernel Oil, Palm Oil, and/or, Soybeans Oil Interesterified, Soybeans Oil Hydrogenated, and/or, Cottonseed Oil Hydrogenated), Chocolate Semisweet (Sugar, Chocolate Liquor Processed With Alkali Dutched, Milk Fat, Soy Lecithin, Emulsifier(s), Vanilla Extract), Milk Non Fat, Eggs Whole, Contains 2% or less of the Following: (, Corn Starch, Eggs Whites, Salt, Sunflower Oil, Soy Lecithin, Flavors Natural, Baking Soda

Rating: 3/10 Stars

## Fig Newton

The fig newton is a very popular kids bar

# Nutrition Facts

Serving Size 31 G
Servings Per Container 13

**Amount Per Serving**

| Calories 110 | Calories from Fat 20 |
|---|---|

| | % Daily Value* |
|---|---|
| **Total Fat** 2 G | 3 |
| Saturated Fat 0 G | 0 |
| Trans Fat 0 G | |
| Monounsaturated Fat 0 G | |
| **Cholesterol** 0 Mg | 0 |
| **Sodium** 130 Mg | 5 |
| **Potassium** 75 Mg | 2 |
| **Total Carbohydrate** 22 G | 7 |
| Dietary Fiber 1 G | 4 |
| Sugars 12 G | |
| **Protein** 1 G | |

| Vitamin A | 0 |
|---|---|
| Vitamin C | 0 |
| Calcium | 2 |

Unbleached Enriched Flour (Wheat Flour, Niacin, Reduced Iron, Thiamine Mononitrate [Vitamin B1], Riboflavin [Vitamin B2], Folic Acid), Figs, High Fructose Corn Syrup, Corn Syrup, Sugar, Soybean Oil, Whey (From Milk), Partially Hydrogenated Cottonseed Oil, Salt, Baking Soda, Cultured Dextrose, Calcium Lactate, Malic Acid, Soy Lecithin, Natural And Artificial Flavor, Sulfur Dioxide Added To Preserve Freshness. Contains: Wheat, Milk, Soy, Sulfites.

3.5/10 stars
High sodium

## Winner

Fiber 1 cookie double choc: why? High fiber, low fat, low sugar, has protein, low calorie, downsides, doesn't taste as good as some of the other cookies, lots of ingredeints.

# Crackers

Crackers are thought to have been invented in 1792 when Theodore Pearson (1753-1817) of Newburyport, Massachusetts, USA, created a pilot-like bread product from just flour and water that he called Pearson's Pilot Bread. It was an instant success with sailors due to its long shelf life.

The real revolutionary moment, however, in the life of the cracker arose in 1801 when a Massachusetts baker, Josiah Bent, burned a batch of biscuits in his brick oven. The crackling noise that he heard from the singed biscuits inspired him to name them crackers. Bent then set out to persuade the world that the product would be a perfect snack food. By 1810, his Boston-area business was thriving, and sometime later Bent sold his business to the National Biscuit Company. By the way the National Biscut Company is now called Nabrisco. Nutritionally, they can be very high in starch but if you choose the right one is could also have high fiber, a good amount of protein and low fat making it a very healthy snack.

# Nabisco Premium Original Saltine Crackers, 16 oz

## Ingredients:

Enriched Flour (Wheat Flour, Niacin, Reduced Iron, Thiamine Mononitrate (Vitamin B1), Riboflavin (Vitamin B2), Folic Acid), Soybean Oil, Salt, High Fructose Corn Syrup, Partially Hydrogenated cottonseed Oil, Malted Barley Flour, Baking Soda, Vegetable Monoglycerides (Emulsifier).

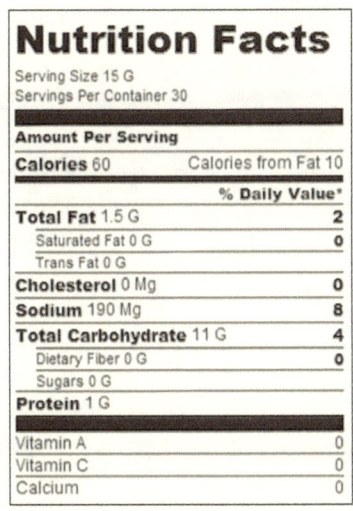

No cholesterol
Low fat
Medium carbohydrates
High sodium
Low protein
No great ingredients
No fiber

Rating: okay

3.5/10 stars

## Sunshine Cheez-It Crackers, 13.7 oz

**Ingredients:** Enriched Flour (Wheat Flour, Niacin, Reduced Iron, Thiamin Mononitrate [Vitamin B1], Riboflavin [Vitamin B2], Folic Acid), Soybean And Palm Oil With Tbhq For Freshness, Skim Milk Cheese (Skim Milk, Whey Protein, Cheese Cultures, Salt, Enzymes, Annatto Extract For Color), Salt, Contains Two Percent Or Less Of Paprika, Yeast, Paprika Oleoresin For Color, Soy Lecithin. Contains Wheat, Milk And Soy Ingredients.

## Nutrition Facts

Serving Size 30 g
Servings Per Container 13

**Amount Per Serving**

| | |
|---|---|
| **Calories** 150 | Calories from Fat 70 |

| | % Daily Value* |
|---|---|
| **Total Fat** 8 g | **12%** |
| Saturated Fat 2 g | **10%** |
| Trans Fat 0 g | |
| **Cholesterol** 0 mg | **0** |
| **Sodium** 250 mg | **10%** |
| **Total Carbohydrate** 17 g | **6%** |
| Dietary Fiber <1 g | **3%** |
| Sugars 0 g | |
| **Protein** 3 g | |

| | |
|---|---|
| Vitamin A | 2% |
| Vitamin C | 0 |
| Calcium | 4% |
| Iron | 6% |

High fat, lots of chemicals, good amount of protein
**Rating:3.5/10 Stars**

## Nabisco Ritz Crackers, 15.1 oz

Unbleached Enriched Flour (Wheat Flour, Niacin, Reduced Iron, Thiamine Mononitrate {Vitamin B1}, Riboflavin {Vitamin B2}, Folic Acid), Soybean Oil, Sugar, Partially Hydrogenated Cottonseed Oil, Salt, Leavening (Baking Soda And/Or Calcium Phosphate), High Fructose Corn Syrup, Soy Lecithin, Malted Barley Flour, Natural Flavor. Contains: Wheat, Soy.

# Nutrition Facts

Serving Size 16 G
Servings Per Container 27

**Amount Per Serving**

| **Calories** 80 | Calories from Fat 40 |
|---|---|
| | **% Daily Value\*** |
| **Total Fat** 4.5 G | **7** |
| Saturated Fat 1 G | **5** |
| Trans Fat 0 G | |
| Monounsaturated Fat 1 G | |
| **Cholesterol** 0 Mg | **0** |
| **Sodium** 105 Mg | **4** |
| **Potassium** 15 Mg | **0** |
| **Total Carbohydrate** 10 G | **3** |
| Dietary Fiber 0 G | **0** |
| Sugars 1 G | |
| **Protein** <1 G | |
| Vitamin A | 0 |
| Vitamin C | 0 |
| Calcium | 2 |

High fat, saturated fat, less sodium, more potassium then average, high fructose corn syrup, hydrogenated cotton seed oil, a little high calorie

**Rating: 2/10 Stars**

# Pepperidge Farm: Goldfish Cheddar Baked Snack Packs Crackers, 12 Oz

Made With Smiles And Unbleached Enriched Wheat Flour [Flour, Niacin, Reduced Iron, Thiamin Mononitrate (Vitamin B1), Riboflavin (Vitamin B2), Folic Acid], Cheddar Cheese [(Pasteurized Cultured Milk, Salt, Enzymes), Annatto], Vegetable Oils (Sunflower, Canola And/Or Soybean), Contains 2 Percent Or Less Of: Salt, Yeast, Sugar, Spices, Autolyzed Yeast, Leavening (Monocalcium Phosphate, Ammonium Bicarbonate, Baking Soda) And Onion Powder.

## Nutrition Facts

Serving Size 30 G
Servings Per Container 28

**Amount Per Serving**

| | |
|---|---|
| **Calories** 140 | Calories from Fat 45 |

| | % Daily Value* |
|---|---|
| **Total Fat** 5 G | **8** |
| Saturated Fat 1 G | **5** |
| Trans Fat 0 G | |
| Monounsaturated Fat 2.5 G | |
| **Cholesterol** <5 Mg | **1** |
| **Sodium** 250 Mg | **10** |
| **Total Carbohydrate** 20 G | **7** |
| Dietary Fiber <1 G | **3** |
| Sugars <1 G | |
| **Protein** 4 G | |

| | |
|---|---|
| Vitamin A | 0 |
| Vitamin C | 0 |
| Calcium | 4 |

High salt, a little high fat, higher protein then most
**Rating: 4.5 Stars**

# Nabisco Triscuit Original Crackers, 13 oz

## Ingredients:

Whole Grain Soft White Wheat, Soybean Oil, Sea Salt, Organic Flax Seeds, Organic Apple Cider Vinegar, Bragg Liquid Aminos (Vegetable Protein from Non-Gmo Soybeans And Purified Water), Organic Dill, Organic Red Chili Peppers.

# Nutrition Facts

Serving Size 28 G
Servings Per Container 13

**Amount Per Serving**

**Calories** 120          Calories from Fat 35

| | % Daily Value* |
|---|---|
| **Total Fat** 4 G | **6** |
| Saturated Fat 0.5 G | **3** |
| Trans Fat 0 G | |
| Polyunsaturated Fat 2 G | |
| Monounsaturated Fat 1 G | |
| **Cholesterol** 0 Mg | **0** |
| **Sodium** 160 Mg | **7** |
| **Potassium** 115 Mg | **3** |
| **Total Carbohydrate** 20 G | **7** |
| Dietary Fiber 3 G | **12** |
| Sugars 0 G | |
| **Protein** 3 G | |
| Vitamin A | 0 |
| Vitamin C | 0 |
| Calcium | 0 |
| Phosphorus | 10 |

**Very wholesome cracker, very few ingredients for a store bought cracker, now for the fats it's a little lower then others and also it has a higher amount of protient and fiber then regular crackers.**

**Rating: 5.5/10 Stars**

# Flackers Dill Flax Seed Crackers, 5 oz, (Pack of 12)

Organic Flax Seeds, Organic Apple Cider Vinegar, Bragg Liquid Aminos (Vegetable Protein from Non-Gmo Soybeans And Purified Water), Organic Dill, Organic Red Chili Peppers.

## Nutrition Facts

Serving Size 25 G
Servings Per Container 6

**Amount Per Serving**

**Calories** 110 · Calories from Fat 70

| | % Daily Value* |
|---|---|
| **Total Fat** 8 G | 12 |
| Saturated Fat 0 G | 0 |
| Trans Fat 0 G | |
| **Cholesterol** 0 Mg | 0 |
| **Sodium** 90 Mg | 4 |
| **Potassium** 0 Mg | 0 |
| **Total Carbohydrate** 8 G | 3 |
| Dietary Fiber 7 G | 27 |
| Sugars 0 G | |
| **Protein** 5 G | |
| Vitamin A | 0 |
| Vitamin C | 0 |
| Calcium | 4 |

Postitives: low carlorie, low sodium, VERY LOW CARBS!, high in protein, higher fats then normal, but redeemed by the fact that most of the fats come from the flax seeds which also provide tons of fiber
**RATING: 8.5 Stars**

# Nabisco Wheat Thins Original Crackers, 10 oz

Whole Grain Wheat Flour, Unbleached Enriched Flour (Wheat Flour, Niacin, Reduced Iron, Thiamine Mononitrate [Vitamin B1], Riboflavin [Vitamin B2], Folic Acid), Soybean Oil, Sugar, Cornstarch, Malt Syrup (From Barley And Corn), Salt, Invert Sugar, Monoglycerides, Leavening (Calcium Phosphate And/Or Baking Soda), Vegetable Color (Annatto Extract, Turmeric Oleoresin). Contains: Wheat. BHT Added To Packaging Material To Preserve Freshness.

# Nutrition Facts

Serving Size 31 G
Servings Per Container 9

**Amount Per Serving**

**Calories** 140      Calories from Fat 45

| | % Daily Value* |
|---|---|
| **Total Fat** 5 G | 8 |
| Saturated Fat 1 G | 5 |
| Trans Fat 0 G | |
| Monounsaturated Fat 1 G | |
| **Cholesterol** 0 Mg | 0 |
| **Sodium** 230 Mg | 10 |
| **Potassium** 60 Mg | 2 |
| **Total Carbohydrate** 22 G | 7 |
| Dietary Fiber 2 G | 8 |
| Sugars 4 G | |
| **Protein** 2 G | |
| Vitamin A | 0 |
| Vitamin C | 0 |
| Calcium | 2 |

Low fat, high sodium, good amount of potassium, medium carbs
**Rating: 4/10 Stars**

## Triscut Whole Wheat Crackers

## Kashi TLC TLC Tasty Little Crackers, Original 7 Grain 9 oz (255 g)

Wheat Flour (Unbleached), Kashi Seven Whole Grains & Sesame Flour (Whole Oats, Hard Red Winter Wheat, Rye, Long Grain Brown Rice, Triticale, Barley, Buckwheat, Sesamum Indicum (Sesame) Oil, Expeller Pressed Sunflower Oil, Evaporated Cane Juice, Toasted Whole Wheat, Toasted Sesame Seeds, Wheat Bran, Co

2% or Less of: Brown Rice Syrup, Stone Ground Whole Wheat Flour, Sea Salt, Malt Extract, Yellow Corn Meal, Millet, Onion Powder, Horseradish Powder, Rice Flour, Malted Barley Flour, Natural Leavenings (Potassium Bicarbonate, Sodium Acid Pyrophosphate, Monocalcium Phosphate, Whey

### Supplement Facts

Serving Size: 15 Crackers (30 g)
Servings Per Container: 8

| Amount per Serving | | |
|---|---|---|
| Calories Total | 130 | |
| from Fat | 30 | |

| Amount per Serving | | % Daily Value+ |
|---|---|---|
| Total Fat | 3 g | 5% |
| Saturated Fat | 0 g | 0% |
| Cholesterol | 0 mg | 0% |
| Sodium | 200 mg | 8% |
| Total Carbohydrate | 22 g | 7% |
| Dietary fiber | 2 g | 8% |
| Sugars | 3 g | |
| Protein | 3 g | |

| | | % Daily Value |
|---|---|---|
| Vitamin A | IU | 0% |
| Vitamin C | mg | 0% |
| Calcium | mg | 2% |
| Iron | mg | 2% |

* Daily Value not established.
+ Percent Daily Values are based on a 2,000 calorie diet. Your daily values may be higher or lower depending on your calorie needs.

Low fat, medium carbs, a lot less fiber then you would guess from the packaging.
Rating: 6/10 Stars

## Wellington Flax Crackers

# Nutrition Facts
Serving Size 7 crackers (30 g)

| Per Serving | % Daily Value* |
|---|---|
| Calories 120 | |
| Calories from Fat 36 | |
| Total Fat 4g | 6% |
| Saturated Fat 0g | 0% |
| Cholesterol 0mg | 0% |
| Sodium 180mg | 8% |
| Carbohydrates 19g | 6% |
| Dietary Fiber 2g | 8% |
| Sugars 2g | |
| Protein 3g | |

Vitamin A 0% · Vitamin C 0%
Calcium 0% · Iron 6%

Organic Wheat Flour, Organic Whole Wheat Flour, Organic Sunflower Oil, Organic Evaporated Cane Juice, Organic Flax Seeds, Organic Cane Syrup, Salt, Sodium Bicarbonate, Organic Wheat Bran, Organic Onion Powder, Enzymes. Contains Wheat. Manufactured In A Facility That Processes Milk, Soy And Sesame Seeds.

Low fat, good amount of protein, low calorie, wholesome ingredients.
Rating: 6.5 stars

# Doctor Kracker

**Nutrition Facts – 6 oz (170g)**

| Serving Size: 8 pieces (28g) | Calories: 120 |
| Servings Per Container: 6 | Calories from Fat: 40 |

| % Daily Value* | | % Daily Value* | | % Daily Value* | |
|---|---|---|---|---|---|
| Total Fat 4.5g | 7% | Total Carbohydrate 14g | 5% | Vitamin A | 0% |
| Saturated Fat 1g | 5% | Dietary Fiber 3g | 12% | Vitamin C | 0% |
| Trans Fat 0g | | Sugars 2g | | Calcium | 3% |
| | | Protein 5g | | Iron | 11% |
| Cholesterol 0mg | 0% | | | | |
| Sodium 145mg | 6% | | | | |

\* Percent Daily Values are based on a 2,000 calorie diet. Your daily values may be higher or lower depending on your caloric needs.

INGREDIENTS: ORGANIC WHOLE SPELT FLOUR, ORGANIC PUMPKIN SEEDS, ORGANIC MILLET, ORGANIC AGAVE SYRUP, ORGANIC SESAME SEEDS, ORGANIC POPPY SEEDS, ORGANIC MOLASSES, ORGANIC FLAXSEEDS, ORGANIC PALM OIL, FILTERED WATER, SEA SALT, ORGANIC WHEAT BRAN, YEAST, ROSEMARY EXTRACT.

Low calorie, low carb, high protein, wholesome ingredeints
Rating: 7/10 Stars

## Winner:

Flacker Flax seed crackers from **Doctor in the Kitchen** have great nutrients, low carbohydrates, high in fiber and protein. Virtually no sugar, delicious, wholesome, higher fat than normal but redeemed by the fact that most of the fats come from the flax seed, which provides tons of fiber.

# Granola Bars

Granola bars are a typical snack that can be a healthy part of any child's lunch box. The problem is that nowadays manufactures are adding too much sugar, salt and fat with not enough fiber and protein, making these bars sometimes more like candy bars then traditional granola bars. In my mind the ideal granola bar would be something with simple ingredients, high fiber and protein with not too high fat and sugar.

# Nature Valley Crunchy Oats 'n Honey Granola Bars, 1.5 oz, 12 count

**Whole Grain Rolled Oats, Sugar, Canola Oil, Crisp Rice With Soy Protein (Rice Flour, Soy Protein Concentrate, Sugar, Malt, Salt), Honey, Brown Sugar Syrup, Salt, Soy Lecithin, Baking Soda, Natural Flavor, Peanut Flour, Almond Flour, Pecan Flour.**

# Nutrition Facts

Serving Size 42 G
Servings Per Container 12

| Amount Per Serving | 2 Bars | 1 Bar |
|---|---|---|
| **Calories** | 180 | 90 |
| Calories from Fat | 50 | 25 |

| | % Daily Value* | |
|---|---|---|
| **Total Fat** 6 G | 9 | 5 |
| Saturated Fat 0.5 G | 3 | 0 |
| Trans Fat 0 G | | |
| **Cholesterol** 0 Mg | 0 | 0 |
| **Sodium** 160 Mg | 7 | 3 |
| **Total Carbohydrate** 29 G | 10 | 5 |
| Sugars 11 G | | |
| **Protein** 4 G | | |

(-) Information is currently not available for this nutrient.

* Percent Daily Values are based on a 2,000 calorie diet. Your daily values may be higher or lower depending on your calorie needs:**

** Percent Daily Values listed below are intended for adults and children over 4 years of age. Foods represented or purported to be for use by infants, children less than 4 years of age, pregnant women, or lactating women shall use the RDI's that are specified for the intended group provided by the FDA.

| | Calories: | 2,000 | 2,500 |
|---|---|---|---|
| Total Fat | Less than | 65g | 80g |
| Sat. Fat | Less than | 20g | 25g |
| Cholesterol | Less than | 300mg | 300mg |
| Sodium | Less than | 2400mg | 2400mg |
| Potassium | | 3500mg | 3500mg |
| Total Carbohydrate | | 300mg | 375mg |
| Dietary Fiber | | 25mg | 30mg |

Calories per gram:

Fat 9 · Carbohydrate 4 · Protein 4

Great ingredeints, high carb, surprisingly no fiber, not a lot of fat for the size and the protein is pretty good too. Rating: 3 /10 Stars

# Nature Valley Sweet & Salty Nut Almond Granola Bars, 1.2 oz, 6 count

(Cultured Whey Almonds, High Maltose Corn Syrup, Rolled Oats, Sugar, High Fructose Corn Syrup, Crisp Rice (Rice Flour, Sugar, Malt, Salt), Palm Kernel Oil, Wheat Flakes (Whole Wheat, Sugar, Salt, Malt), Fructose, Canola Oil, Water, Yogurt Powder Protein Concentrate, Cultured Skim Milk, Yogurt Cultures), Maltodextrin, Salt, Nonfat Milk, Soy Lecithin, Color Added, Honey, Natural Flavor, Baking Soda, Sunflower Meal, Peanut Flour, Mixed Tocopherols Added To Retain Freshness. Contains Almond, Wheat, Milk, Soy, Sunflower And Peanut Ingredients.

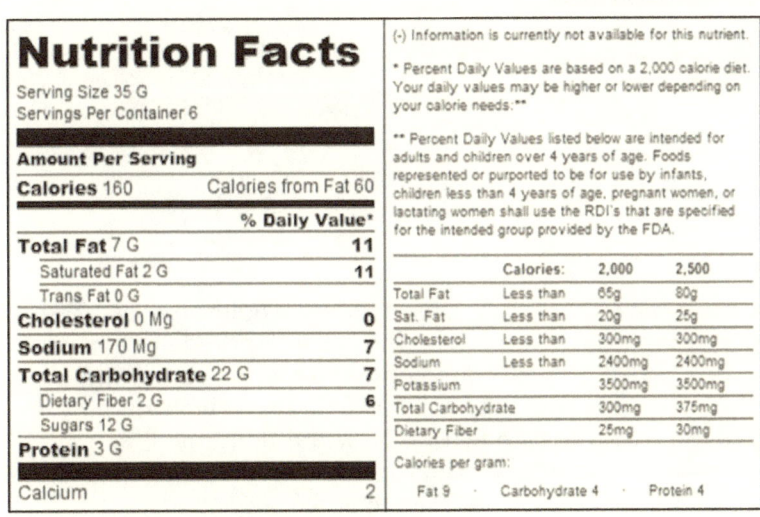

## Nutrition Facts

Serving Size 35 G
Servings Per Container 6

**Amount Per Serving**

**Calories** 160 — Calories from Fat 60

| | % Daily Value* |
|---|---|
| **Total Fat** 7 G | 11 |
| Saturated Fat 2 G | 11 |
| Trans Fat 0 G | |
| **Cholesterol** 0 Mg | 0 |
| **Sodium** 170 Mg | 7 |
| **Total Carbohydrate** 22 G | 7 |
| Dietary Fiber 2 G | 6 |
| Sugars 12 G | |
| **Protein** 3 G | |
| Calcium | 2 |

(-) Information is currently not available for this nutrient.

* Percent Daily Values are based on a 2,000 calorie diet. Your daily values may be higher or lower depending on your calorie needs:**

** Percent Daily Values listed below are intended for adults and children over 4 years of age. Foods represented or purported to be for use by infants, children less than 4 years of age, pregnant women, or lactating women shall use the RDI's that are specified for the intended group provided by the FDA.

| | Calories: | 2,000 | 2,500 |
|---|---|---|---|
| Total Fat | Less than | 65g | 80g |
| Sat. Fat | Less than | 20g | 25g |
| Cholesterol | Less than | 300mg | 300mg |
| Sodium | Less than | 2400mg | 2400mg |
| Potassium | | 3500mg | 3500mg |
| Total Carbohydrate | | 300mg | 375mg |
| Dietary Fiber | | 25mg | 30mg |

Calories per gram:
Fat 9 · Carbohydrate 4 · Protein 4

- High in fat

Rating: 3 stars

# Quacker Chewy Bars

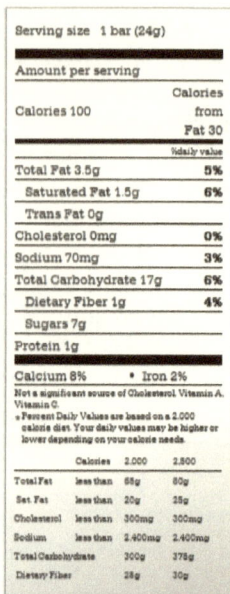

**Ingredients**

GRANOLA (WHOLE GRAIN ROLLED OATS, BROWNSUGAR, CRISP RICE [RICE FLOUR, SUGAR, SALT, MALTED BARLEY EXTRACT],WHOLE GRAIN ROLLED WHEAT, SOYBEAN OIL, DRIED COCONUT, WHOLE WHEATFLOUR, SODIUM BICARBONATE, SOY LECITHIN, CARAMEL COLOR, NONFAT DRYMILK), SEMISWEET CHOCOLATE CHIPS (SUGAR, CHOCOLATE LIQUOR, COCOABUTTER, SOY LECITHIN, VANILLA EXTRACT), CORN SYRUP, BROWN RICE CRISP(WHOLE GRAIN BROWN RICE, SUGAR, MALTED BARLEY FLOUR, SALT), INVERTSUGAR, SUGAR, CORN SYRUP SOLIDS, GLYCERIN, SOYBEAN OIL. CONTAINS 2% OR LESS OF SORBITOL,CALCIUM CARBONATE, SALT, WATER, SOY LECITHIN, MOLASSES, NATURAL ANDARTIFICIAL FLAVOR, BHT (PRESERVATIVE), CITRIC ACID.

*The nutrition facts of some club pack offerings may differ. Check your label.

CONTAINS WHEAT, COCONUT, SOY AND MILK INGREDIENTS.

MAY CONTAIN TRACES OF PEANUT AND OTHER TREE NUTS.

I have got to say, this is a very wholesome bar. The first ingredient is granola, the second ingredient is crisp rice and the third ingredient whole grain rolled wheat! Also I think this may be our first snack with no HFCS (high fructose corn syrup). Now the nutritional facts on this aren't so hot. There are 16 grams of real carbs (that means the carbs other than fiber are sugar and starch). It also has 1.5 grams of pure saturated fat.

Rating: 4.5/10 Stars

# QUAKER® CHEWY GRANOLA BARS

## PEANUT BUTTERCHOCOLATE CHIP

| Serving size 1 Bar (24g) | | |
|---|---|---|
| **Amount per serving** | | |
| | | Calories |
| Calories 100 | | from Fat 25 |
| | | %daily value |
| Total Fat 3g | | 4% |
| Saturated Fat 1g | | 4% |
| Trans Fat 0g | | |
| Sodium 95mg | | 4% |
| Total Carbohydrate 17g | | 6% |
| Dietary Fiber 1g | | 4% |
| Sugars 7g | | |
| Protein 2g | | |
| Calcium 10% | • | Iron 2% |

Not a significant source of Cholesterol, Vitamin A, Vitamin C.

*Percent Daily Values are based on a 2,000 calorie diet. Your daily values may be higher or lower depending on your calorie needs.*

| | Calories | 2,000 | 2,500 |
|---|---|---|---|
| Total Fat | less than | 65g | 80g |
| Sat Fat | less than | 20g | 25g |
| Cholesterol | less than | 300mg | 300mg |
| Sodium | less than | 2,400mg | 2,400mg |
| Total Carbohydrate | | 300g | 375g |
| Dietary Fiber | | 25g | 30g |

**Ingredients**
GRANOLA (WHOLE GRAIN ROLLED OATS, BROWN SUGAR, CRISP RICE [RICE FLOUR, SUGAR, SALT, MALTED BARLEY EXTRACT], WHOLE GRAIN ROLLED WHEAT, SOYBEAN OIL, WHOLE WHEAT FLOUR, SODIUM BICARBONATE, SOY LECITHIN, CARAMEL COLOR, NONFAT DRY MILK), CORN SYRUP, BROWN RICE CRISP (WHOLE GRAIN BROWN RICE, SUGAR, MALTED BARLEY FLOUR, SALT), PEANUT BUTTER SPREAD (PEANUTS, SUGAR, PALM OIL, SALT), SEMISWEET CHOCOLATE CHIPS (SUGAR, CHOCOLATE LIQUOR, COCOA BUTTER, SOY LECITHIN, VANILLA EXTRACT), INVERT SUGAR, PEANUT FLAVORED CHIPS (SUGAR, PALM KERNEL AND PALM OIL, PARTIALLY DEFATTED PEANUT FLOUR, LACTOSE, DRY WHEY, DEXTROSE, CORN SYRUP SOLIDS, SOY LECITHIN, SALT, VANILLIN [ARTIFICIAL FLAVOR]), CORN SYRUP SOLIDS, GLYCERIN. CONTAINS 2% OR LESS OF CALCIUM CARBONATE, SORBITOL, SALT, WATER, NATURAL AND ARTIFICIAL FLAVOR, BHT (PRESERVATIVE), CITRIC ACID.

*The nutrition facts of some club pack offerings may differ. Check your label.

**CONTAINS WHEAT, SOY, PEANUT AND MILK INGREDIENTS.**

**MAY CONTAIN TRACES OF TREE NUTS.**

Rating: 3/10 stars

*Zain Naqvi*

# QUAKER® CHEWY DIPPS GRANOLA BARS

**Nutrition Facts**

Serving size 1 Bar (30 g)
Servings Per Container see table

| Amount per serving | |
|---|---|
| Calories 150 | Calories from Fat 60 |

| | %Daily Value* |
|---|---|
| **Total Fat** 7g | **11%** |
| Saturated Fat 3.5g | **18%** |
| Trans Fat 0.5g | |
| Polyunsaturated Fat 1g | |
| Monounsaturated Fat 1.5g | |
| **Cholesterol** 0mg | **0%** |
| **Sodium** 85mg | **4%** |
| **Total Carbohydrate** 20g | **7%** |
| Dietary Fiber 1g | **4%** |
| Sugars 11g | |
| Sugar Alcohol 1g | |
| Other Carbohydrate 7g | |
| **Protein** 2g | |
| Iron | **2%** |

*Not a significant source of vitamin A, vitamin C and calcium

*Percent Daily Values are based on a 2,000 calorie diet. Your daily values may be higher or lower depending on your calorie needs

| | Calories | 2,000 | 2,500 |
|---|---|---|---|
| Total Fat | less than | 65g | 80g |
| Sat. Fat | less than | 20g | 25g |
| Cholesterol | less than | 300mg | 300mg |
| Sodium | less than | 2,400mg | 2,400mg |
| Total Carbohydrate | | 300g | 375g |
| Dietary Fiber | | 25g | 30g |

**Ingredients**

Granola (whole grain rolled oats, whole grain rolled wheat, sugar, sunflower oil, high fructose corn syrup, molasses, dried coconut, honey, sodium bicarbonate, natural flavor, whey protein concentrate), sugar, peanuts, partially hydrogenated palm kernel, palm oil and soybean oil, crisp rice (rice flour, sugar, barley malt, salt), corn syrup solids, corn syrup, high fructose corn syrup, whey, hydrogenated vegetable oil (cottonseed and soybean), brown sugar, dextrose, lactose, glycerin, cocoa, cocoa processed with alkali, sorbitol, salt, milkfat, soy lecithin, natural and artificial flavor, glyceryl lacto esters of fatty acids, BHT (preservative).

**CONTAINS WHEAT, COCONUT, MILK, PEANUT AND SOY INGREDIENTS. MAY CONTAIN TRACES OF OTHER TREE NUTS.**

Rating: 3.5/10 stars

# QUAKER® CHEWY DIPPS GRANOLA BARS

## PEANUT BUTTER CHOCOLATE

Serving size 1 Bar (31g)
Servings Per Container 6

| Amount per serving | |
|---|---|
| | Calories from Fat 50 |
| Calories 140 | |

| | %daily value* |
|---|---|
| Total Fat 6g | 10% |
| Saturated Fat 4.5g | 21% |
| Trans Fat 0g | |
| Polyunsaturated Fat 0g | |
| Monounsaturated Fat 1g | |
| Cholesterol 0mg | 0% |
| Sodium 65mg | 3% |
| Total Carbohydrate 21g | 7% |
| Dietary Fiber 1g | 4% |
| Sugars 12g | |
| Sugar Alcohol 1g | |
| Protein 2g | |
| Iron | 2% |

Not a significant source of Vitamin A, Vitamin C and Calcium.

*Percent Daily Values are based on a 2,000 calorie diet. Your daily values may be higher or lower depending on your calorie needs:

| | Calories | 2,000 | 2,500 |
|---|---|---|---|
| Total Fat | less than | 65g | 80g |
| Sat. Fat | less than | 20g | 25g |
| Cholesterol | less than | 300mg | 300mg |
| Sodium | less than | 2,400mg | 2,400mg |
| Total Carbohydrate | | 300g | 375g |
| Dietary Fiber | | 25g | 30g |

**Ingredients**
GRANOLA (WHOLE GRAIN ROLLED OATS, WHOLE GRAIN ROLLED WHEAT, SUGAR, SUNFLOWER OIL, HIGH FRUCTOSE CORN SYRUP, MOLASSES, DRIED COCONUT, HONEY, SODIUM BICARBONATE, NATURAL FLAVOR, WHEY PROTEIN CONCENTRATE), SUGAR, PALM KERNEL AND PALM OIL, CRISP RICE (RICE FLOUR, SUGAR, BARLEY MALT, SALT), SEMISWEET CHOCOLATE CHIPS (SUGAR, CHOCOLATE LIQUOR, COCOA BUTTER, SOY LECITHIN, VANILLA EXTRACT), CORN SYRUP, PARTIALLY DEFATTED PEANUT FLOUR, HIGH FRUCTOSE CORN SYRUP, CORN SYRUP SOLIDS, BROWN SUGAR, GLYCERIN, LACTOSE, PARTIALLY HYDROGENATED SOYBEAN OIL*, WHEY POWDER, DEXTROSE, SORBITOL, COCOA (PROCESSED WITH ALKALI), SALT, SOY LECITHIN, ARTIFICIAL FLAVOR, BHT (PRESERVATIVE), CITRIC ACID, WATER.

*ADDS A DIETARILY INSIGNIFICANT AMOUNT OF TRANS FAT

**CONTAINS WHEAT, COCONUT, MILK, SOY AND PEANUT INGREDIENTS.
MAY CONTAIN TRACES OF OTHER TREE NUTS.**

Rating: 4.5/10 Stars

## *QUAKER® CHEWY® YOGURT GRANOLA BAR*

## **VANILLA**

### Nutrition Facts

Serving size 1 bar (35g)
Servings Per Container

Amount per serving

| | Calories |
|---|---|
| Calories 150 | from Fat 40 |

| | %daily value* |
|---|---|
| Total Fat 4.5g | 7% |
| Saturated Fat 2.5g | 12% |
| Trans Fat 0g | |
| Polyunsaturated Fat 0.5g | |
| Monounsaturated Fat 1g | |
| Cholesterol 0mg | 0% |
| Sodium 115mg | 5% |
| Total Carbohydrate 25g | 8% |
| Dietary Fiber 1g | 5% |
| Sugars 11g | |
| Sugar Alcohol 2g | |
| Protein 2g | |

Calcium 10% • Iron 2%

Not a significant source of
vitamin A and vitamin C.
*Percent Daily Values are based
on a 2,000 calorie diet. Your
daily values may be higher or
lower depending on your calorie
needs:

| | Calories | 2,000 | 2,500 |
|---|---|---|---|
| Total Fat | Less than | 65g | 80g |
| Sat Fat | Less than | 20g | 25g |
| Cholesterol | Less than | 300mg | 300mg |
| Sodium | Less than | 2,400mg | 2,400mg |
| Total Carbohydrate | | 300g | 375g |
| Dietary Fiber | | 25g | 30g |

**Ingredients**

GRANOLA (WHOLE GRAIN ROLLED OATS, WHOLE GRAIN ROLLED WHEAT, BROWN SUGAR, SUNFLOWER OIL, INVERT SUGAR, DRIED COCONUT, HONEY, SODIUM BICARBONATE, NATURAL FLAVOR, WHEY AND WHEY PROTEIN CONCENTRATE), YOGURT FLAVORED COATING (SUGAR, PALM KERNEL AND PALM OIL, WHEY PROTEIN CONCENTRATE, DRIED YOGURT (HEAT-TREATED AFTER CULTURING) [CULTURED NONFAT DRY MILK, LACTIC ACID, CITRIC ACID], SOY LECITHIN, NATURAL FLAVOR, ARTIFICIAL COLOR, CITRIC ACID, SALT), CORN SYRUP, INVERT SUGAR, BROWN RICE CRISP (WHOLE GRAIN BROWN RICE FLOUR, SUGAR, MALTED BARLEY FLOUR, SALT), BROWN SUGAR, GLYCERIN, VEGETABLE SHORTENING (CANOLA OIL, PALM AND PALM KERNEL OILS), CORN FLAKES (MILLED CORN, SUGAR, SALT, MALTED BARLEY EXTRACT), WHEY MINERAL CONCENTRATE, OAT FLOUR, RICE FLOUR, CORN SYRUP SOLIDS, SORBITOL, SALT, SUGAR, MODIFIED FOOD STARCH, SOY LECITHIN, NATURAL FLAVOR, MALTED BARLEY FLOUR, SODIUM BICARBONATE, BHT (A PRESERVATIVE), CITRIC ACID, WATER.

**CONTAINS WHEAT, COCONUT, MILK AND SOY INGREDIENTS.**

**MAY CONTAIN TRACES OF PEANUT AND OTHER TREE NUTS.**
31281-1

The yogurt granola bars are basically the regular granola bars dipped in yoghurt. Yoghurt is healthy, but it is best eaten fresh so you know you are getting real yoghurt. Also adding it onto a granola bar adds unneeded calorie.

Rating: 5/10 Stars

# QUAKER® CHEWY® YOGURT GRANOLA BAR

## STRAWBERRY

## Nutrition Facts

Serving size 1 bar (35g)
Servings Per Container

| Amount per serving | |
|---|---|
| | Calories |
| Calories 150 | from |
| | Fat 40 |

| | %daily value* |
|---|---|
| **Total Fat 4.5g** | **7%** |
| Saturated Fat 2.5g | 12% |
| Trans Fat 0g | |
| Polyunsaturated Fat 0.5g | |
| Monounsaturated Fat 1g | |
| **Cholesterol** 0mg | **0%** |
| **Sodium** 115mg | **5%** |
| **Total Carbohydrate** 25g | **8%** |
| Dietary Fiber 1g | 5% |
| Sugars 11g | |
| Sugar Alcohol 2g | |
| **Protein** 2g | |

Calcium 10%  •  Iron 2%

Not a significant source of vitamin A and vitamin C.

*Percent Daily Values are based on a 2,000 calorie diet. Your daily values may be higher or lower depending on your calorie needs:

| | Calories | 2,000 | 2,500 |
|---|---|---|---|
| Total Fat | Less than | 65g | 80g |
| Sat. Fat | Less than | 20g | 25g |
| Cholesterol | Less than | 300mg | 300mg |
| Sodium | Less than | 2,400mg | 2,400mg |
| Total Carbohydrate | | 300g | 375g |
| Dietary Fiber | | 25g | 30g |

**Ingredients**
GRANOLA (WHOLE GRAIN ROLLED OATS, WHOLE GRAIN ROLLED WHEAT, BROWN SUGAR, SUNFLOWER OIL, INVERT SUGAR, DRIED COCONUT, HONEY, SODIUM BICARBONATE, NATURAL FLAVOR, WHEY AND WHEY PROTEIN CONCENTRATE), YOGURT FLAVORED COATING (SUGAR, PALM KERNEL AND PALM OIL, WHEY PROTEIN CONCENTRATE, DRIED YOGURT [HEATTREATED AFTER CULTURING] [CULTURED NONFAT DRY MILK, LACTIC ACID, CITRIC ACID], SOY LECITHIN, NATURAL FLAVOR, ARTIFICIAL COLOR, CITRIC ACID, SALT), CORN SYRUP, INVERT SUGAR, BROWN RICE CRISP (WHOLE GRAIN BROWN RICE FLOUR, SUGAR, MALTED BARLEY FLOUR, SALT), BROWN SUGAR, GLYCERIN, VEGETABLE SHORTENING (CANOLA OIL, PALM AND PALM KERNEL OILS), CORN FLAKES (MILLED CORN, SUGAR, SALT, MALTED BARLEY EXTRACT), WHEY MINERAL CONCENTRATE, OAT FLOUR, RICE FLOUR, SWEETENED DRIED STRAWBERRIES (GLUCOSE SYRUP, STRAWBERRIES, FRUCTOSE, MODIFIED POTATO STARCH, SODIUM ALGINATE), CORN SYRUP SOLIDS, SORBITOL, SALT, SUGAR, MODIFIED FOOD STARCH, SOY LECITHIN, NATURAL FLAVOR, MALTED BARLEY FLOUR, SODIUM BICARBONATE, BHT (A PRESERVATIVE), CITRIC ACID, WATER.

**CONTAINS WHEAT, COCONUT, MILK AND SOY INGREDIENTS.**

**MAY CONTAIN TRACES OF PEANUT AND OTHER TREE NUTS.**
31280-1

Rating 5/10 Stars

## Strawberry Nutri-Grain bar

# Nutrition Facts
# Valeur nutritive
Per 1 bar (37 g) / pour 1 barre (37 g)

| Amount<br>Teneur | % Daily Value<br>% valeur quotidienne |
|---|---|
| **Calories / Calories** 130 | |
| **Fat / Lipides** 3 g | **5 %** |
| Saturated / saturés 0.5 g<br>+ Trans / trans 0 g | **3 %** |
| **Cholesterol / Cholestérol** 0 mg | **0 %** |
| **Sodium / Sodium** 100 mg | **4 %** |
| **Potassium / Potassium** 85 mg | **2 %** |
| **Carbohydrate / Glucides** 25 g | **8 %** |
| Fibre / Fibres 2 g | **8 %** |
| Sugars / Sucres 13 g | |
| **Protein / Protéines** 2 g | |
| Vitamin A / Vitamine A | 0 % |
| Vitamin C / Vitamine C | 0 % |
| Calcium / Calcium | 2 % |
| Iron / Fer | 10 % |

Rating: 3.5/10

All of the nutri-Grain bars are very similar in terms of nutrition. Although they advertise lots of fiber, one quick look at the nutrition facts can tell us that this isn't the case. Also this isn't a very natural bar and we can tell by the ingredient list that there are a lot of chemicals in it.

# Kashi Trail mix bar

## Nutrition

| | |
|---|---|
| Serving Size | 1 Bar |
| Calories | 140 |
| Total Fat | 5 g |
| Sodium | 95 mg |
| Fiber | 4 g |
| Sugar | 6 g |
| Protein | 6 g |
| Whole Grains | 11 g |

See entire nutrition panel >>

## Ingredients

Rolled Whole Grain Blend (Hard Red Wheat, Oats, Rye, Triticale, Barley), Roasted Salted Whole Almonds, Brown Rice Syrup, Soy Protein Isolate, Dried Cane Syrup, Soy Grits, Chicory Root Fiber, Raisins, Sunflower Seeds, Cane Syrup, Cranberries, Vegetable Glycerin, Corn Flour, Honey, Rice Starch, Expeller Pressed Canola Oil, Oat Fiber, Evaporated Salt, Natural Flavors, Molasses, Kashi Seven Whole Grains & Sesame Flour (Whole: Oats, Hard Red Wheat, Rye, Brown Rice, Triticale, Barley, Buckwheat, Sesame Seeds), Sunflower Oil, Soy Lecithin, Peanut Flour, Whey Protein Isolate.

## Allergens

Contains Wheat, Almond, Soy, Peanut And Milk Ingredients. May Contain Other Tree Nuts.

Really wholesome, lots of nutrients
Rating: 8/10 Stars

# Kashi Chewy Granola dark mocha almond

## Nutrition

| | |
|---|---|
| Serving Size | 1 Bar |
| Calories | 130 |
| Total Fat | 3.5 g |
| Sodium | 90 mg |
| Fiber | 4 g |
| Sugar | 6 g |
| Protein | 6 g |
| Whole Grains | 12 g |

See entire nutrition panel >>

## Ingredients

Rolled Whole Grain Blend (Hard Red Wheat, Oats, Rye, Triticale, Barley), Brown Rice Syrup, Roasted Salted Whole Almonds, Soy Protein Isolate, Dark Chocolate (Cane Syrup, Chocolate Liquor, Cocoa Butter, Soy Lecithin, Vanilla), Soy Grits, Dried Cane Syrup, Chicory Root Fiber, Cane Syrup, Cocoa, Corn Flour, Honey, Rice Starch, Expeller Pressed Canola Oil, Natural Coffee Extract, Vegetable Glycerin, Natural Flavors, Oat Fiber, Nonfat Milk, Kashi Seven Whole Grains & Sesame Flour (Whole: Oats, Hard Red Wheat, Rye, Brown Rice, Triticale, Barley, Buckwheat, Sesame Seeds), Evaporated Salt, Soy Lecithin, Peanut Flour

## Allergens

Contains Wheat, Almond, Soy, Milk And Peanut Ingredients. May Contain Other Tree Nuts.

Really wholesome, lots of nutrients
Rating: 8/10 Stars

# Quacker Chewy Smores

Ingredients
GRANOLA (WHOLE GRAIN ROLLED OATS, BROWN SUGAR, CRISP RICE [RICE FLOUR, SUGAR, SALT, MALTED BARLEY EXTRACT], WHOLE GRAIN ROLLED WHEAT, SOYBEAN OIL, WHOLE WHEAT FLOUR, SODIUM BICARBONATE, SOY LECITHIN, CARAMEL COLOR, NONFAT DRY MILK), CORN SYRUP, SEMISWEET CHOCOLATE CHIPS (SUGAR, CHOCOLATE LIQUOR, COCOA BUTTER, SOY LECITHIN, VANILLA EXTRACT), BROWN RICE CRISP (WHOLE GRAIN BROWN RICE, SUGAR, MALTED BARLEY FLOUR, SALT), SUGAR, GRAHAM COOKIE PIECES (SUGAR, WHEAT FLOUR, CANOLA OIL, HONEY, SODIUM BICARBONATE, SALT, SOY LECITHIN, NATURAL FLAVOR), DEHYDRATED MARSHMALLOWS (SUGAR, CORN SYRUP, MODIFIED FOOD STARCH, GELATIN, NATURAL AND ARTIFICIAL FLAVOR, SODIUM HEXAMETAPHOSPHATE, BLUE 1), CORN SYRUP SOLIDS, INVERT SUGAR, GLYCERIN. CONTAINS 2% OR LESS OF SOYBEAN OIL, SORBITOL, CALCIUM CARBONATE, SALT, WATER, MOLASSES, SOY LECITHIN, NATURAL AND ARTIFICIAL FLAVOR, CREAMED COCONUT, BHT (PRESERVATIVE), CITRIC ACID.

Serving Size 1 Bar (24 g)
Servings Per Container 8

**Amount per serving**

**Calories** 100 — Calories from Fat 20

| | %Daily Value* |
|---|---|
| **Total Fat** 2g | 3% |
| Saturated Fat 0.5g | 3% |
| Trans Fat 0g | |
| Polyunsaturated Fat 0.5g | |
| Monounsaturated Fat 0.5g | |
| **Cholesterol** 0mg | 0% |
| **Sodium** 75mg | 3% |
| **Total Carbohydrate** 19g | 6% |
| Dietary Fiber 1g | 3% |
| Sugars 8g | |
| Sugar Alcohol 1g | |
| **Protein** 1g | |
| Calcium | 8% |
| Iron | 2% |

Not a significant source of vitamin A, vitamin C.

* Percent Daily Values are based on a 2,000 calorie diet. Your daily values may be higher or lower depending on your calorie needs:

| | | Calories | 2,000 | 2,500 |
|---|---|---|---|---|
| Total Fat | less than | | 65g | 80g |
| Sat Fat | less than | | 20g | 25g |
| Cholesterol | less than | | 300mg | 300mg |
| Sodium | less than | | 2,400mg | 2,400mg |
| Total Carbohydrate | | | 300g | 375g |
| Dietary Fiber | | | 25g | 30g |

Rating 5/10 Stars

# Chocolate dipped bar chocolate chip

Ingredients
GRANOLA (WHOLE GRAIN
ROLLED OATS, WHOLE GRAIN
ROLLED WHEAT, BROWN
SUGAR, SUNFLOWER OIL, HIGH
FRUCTOSE CORN SYRUP, DRIED
UNSWEETENED COCONUT,
HONEY, SODIUM BICARBONATE,
NATURAL FLAVOR, WHEY
PROTEIN CONCENTRATE), SUGAR,
PARTIALLY HYDROGENATED
PALM KERNEL AND PALM OIL*,
CRISP RICE (RICE FLOUR, SUGAR,
BARLEY MALT, SALT), NONFAT
MILK, CORN SYRUP, SEMISWEET
CHOCOLATE CHIPS (SUGAR,
CHOCOLATE LIQUOR, COCOA
BUTTER, SOY LECITHIN, VANILLA
EXTRACT), HIGH FRUCTOSE
CORN SYRUP, BROWN SUGAR,
CORN SYRUP SOLIDS, GLYCERIN,
DRIED WHOLE MILK, PARTIALLY
HYDROGENATED SOYBEAN OIL*,
COCOA PROCESSED WITH ALKALI,
COCOA, SORBITOL, SOY LECITHIN,
SALT, NATURAL AND ARTIFICIAL
FLAVOR, GLYCERYL LACTO
ESTERS OF FATTY ACIDS, BHT
(PRESERVATIVE), CITRIC ACID.
*ADDS A DIETARILY
INSIGNIFICANT AMOUNT OF
TRANS FAT

Serving size   1 Bar (31g)

Amount per serving

|  | Calories |
|---|---|
| Calories 140 | from Fat50 |

| | %daily value |
|---|---|
| Total Fat 6g | 9% |
| Saturated Fat 4g | 20% |
| Trans Fat 0g | |
| Sodium 80mg | 3% |
| Total Carbohydrate 22g | 7% |
| Dietary Fiber 1g | 4% |
| Sugars 12g | |
| Protein 2g | |

Calcium 2%      •   Iron 2%

Not a significant source of
Cholesterol, Vitamin A, Vitamin
C.

*Percent Daily Values are based
on a 2,000 calorie diet. Your
daily values may be higher or
lower depending on your calorie
needs.

| | Calories | 2,000 | 2,800 |
|---|---|---|---|
| Total Fat | less than | 65g | 80g |
| Sat Fat | less than | 20g | 25g |
| Cholesterol | less than | 300mg | 300mg |
| Sodium | less than | 2,400mg | 2,400mg |
| Total Carbohydrate | | 300g | 375g |
| Dietary Fiber | | 25g | 30g |

Rating: 3.5/10

# QUAKER® CHEWY DIPPS GRANOLA BARS

## CARAMEL NUT

Serving size 1 Bar (31g)
Servings Per Container 8

Amount per serving

| | Calories |
|---|---|
| Calories 140 | from |
| | Fat 50 |

| | %daily value |
|---|---|
| Total Fat 6g | 9% |
| Saturated Fat 3.5g | 18% |
| Trans Fat 0g | |
| Polyunsaturated Fat 0.5g | |
| Sodium 65mg | 3% |
| Total Carbohydrate 21g | 7% |
| Dietary Fiber 1g | 3% |
| Sugars 13g | |
| Protein 2g | |

| | |
|---|---|
| Calcium | 2% |
| Iron | 2% |

Not a significant source of Cholesterol, Vitamin A, Vitamin C.

*Percent Daily Values are based on a 2,000 calorie diet. Your daily values may be higher or lower depending on your calorie needs.

| | Calories | 2,000 | 2,500 |
|---|---|---|---|
| Total Fat | less than | 65g | 80g |
| Sat Fat | less than | 20g | 25g |
| Cholesterol | less than | 300mg | 300mg |
| Sodium | less than | 2,400mg | 2,400mg |
| Total Carbohydrate | | 300g | 375g |
| Dietary Fiber | | 25g | 30g |

### Ingredients

CARAMEL (GLUCOSE, SUGAR, PALM OIL, SKIM MILK, GLYCERIN, BUTTER [CREAM, SALT], MODIFIED FOOD STARCH, WHEY, SALT, MONO AND DIGLYCERIDES, SOY LECITHIN), GRANOLA (WHOLE GRAIN ROLLED OATS, WHOLE GRAIN ROLLED WHEAT, BROWN SUGAR, SUNFLOWER OIL, HIGH FRUCTOSE CORN SYRUP, DRIED UNSWEETENED COCONUT, HONEY, SODIUM BICARBONATE, NATURAL FLAVOR, WHEY PROTEIN CONCENTRATE), SUGAR, PARTIALLY HYDROGENATED PALM KERNEL AND PALM OIL, CRISP RICE (RICE FLOUR, SUGAR, BARLEY MALT EXTRACT, SALT), NONFAT MILK, CORN SYRUP, PEANUTS, HIGH FRUCTOSE CORN SYRUP, BROWN SUGAR, CORN SYRUP SOLIDS, DRIED WHOLE MILK, GLYCERIN, COCOA PROCESSED WITH ALKALI, COCOA, CANOLA OIL, PALM OIL AND PALM KERNEL OILS, SORBITOL, SOY LECITHIN, SALT, NATURAL AND ARTIFICIAL FLAVOR, GLYCERYL LACTO ESTERS OF FATTY ACIDS, BHT (PRESERVATIVE), CITRIC ACID, WATER.

CONTAINS WHEAT, COCONUT, MILK, PEANUT AND SOY INGREDIENTS.
MAY CONTAIN TRACES OF TREE NUTS.

Rating 4/10 Stars

# QUAKER® CHEWY DIPPS GRANOLA BARS

## PEANUT BUTTER

| Nutrition Facts | |
|---|---|
| Serving size 1 Bar (30g) | |
| Servings Per Container 8 | |

| Amount per serving | |
|---|---|
| | Calories |
| Calories 150 | from |
| | Fat 60 |

| | %daily value |
|---|---|
| Total Fat 7g | 11% |
| Saturated Fat 3.5g | 17% |
| Trans Fat 0.5g | |
| Sodium 105mg | 4% |
| Total Carbohydrate 19g | 6% |
| Dietary Fiber 1g | 4% |
| Sugars 10g | |
| Protein 3g | |

| Calcium 2% | Iron 2% |
|---|---|

Not a significant source of Cholesterol, Vitamin A, Vitamin C.

*Percent Daily Values are based on a 2,000 calorie diet. Your daily values may be higher or lower depending on your calorie needs.

| | Calories | 2,000 | 2,500 |
|---|---|---|---|
| Total Fat | less than | 65g | 80g |
| Sat Fat | less than | 20g | 25g |
| Cholesterol | less than | 300mg | 300mg |
| Sodium | less than | 2,400mg | 2,400mg |
| Total Carbohydrate | | 300g | 375g |
| Dietary Fiber | | 25g | 30g |

**Ingredients**
GRANOLA (WHOLE GRAIN ROLLED OATS, WHOLE GRAIN ROLLED WHEAT, BROWN SUGAR, SUNFLOWER OIL, HIGH FRUCTOSE CORN SYRUP, DRIED UNSWEETENED COCONUT, HONEY, SODIUM BICARBONATE, NATURAL FLAVOR, WHEY PROTEIN CONCENTRATE), SUGAR, PEANUTS, PARTIALLY HYDROGENATED PALM KERNEL AND PALM OIL*, CRISP RICE (RICE FLOUR, SUGAR, BARLEY MALT EXTRACT, SALT), NONFAT MILK, CORN SYRUP SOLIDS, CORN SYRUP, HIGH FRUCTOSE CORN SYRUP, HYDROGENATED VEGETABLE OIL* (COTTONSEED AND SOYBEAN OIL), CITRIC ACID, BROWN SUGAR, DEXTROSE, DRIED WHOLE MILK, GLYCERIN, COCOA PROCESSED WITH ALKALI, COCOA, SORBITOL, HYDROGENATED SOYBEAN OIL*, HYDROGENATED PALM OIL* (PALM OIL AND/OR FRACTIONATED PALM OIL), SALT, SOY LECITHIN, NATURAL AND ARTIFICIAL FLAVOR, GLYCERYL LACTO ESTERS OF FATTY ACIDS, BH (PRESERVATIVE).*ADDS A DIETARILY INSIGNIFICANT AMOUNT OF TRANS FAT

**CONTAINS WHEAT, COCONUT, MILK, PEANUT AND SOY INGREDIENTS.**
**MAY CONTAIN TRACES OF TREE NUTS.**

Rating: 4.5/10

# QUAKER® CHEWY DIPPS GRANOLA BARS

## DARK CHOCOLATEY

| Serving size 1 Bar (31g) | |
|---|---|
| Serving Per Container 6 | |

| Amount per serving | |
|---|---|
| | Calories |
| Calories 140 | from |
| | Fat 45 |

| | %daily value |
|---|---|
| Total Fat 5g | 8% |
| Saturated Fat 4g | 19% |
| Trans Fat 0g | |
| Polyunsaturated Fat 0g | |
| Monounsaturated Fat 1 g | |
| Cholesterol 0mg | 0% |
| Sodium 55mg | 2% |
| Total Carbohydrate 23g | 8% |
| Dietary Fiber 1g | 4% |
| Sugars 13g | |
| Sugar Alcohol 1g | |
| Other Carbohydrate 8g | |
| Protein 2g | |
| Vitamin A 0g | |
| Vitamin C 0g | |
| Calcium 0% | |
| Iron 2% | |

*Percent Daily Values are based on a 2,000 calorie diet. Your daily values may be higher or lower depending on your calorie needs.

| | Calories | 2,000 | 3,000 |
|---|---|---|---|
| Total Fat | less than | 65g | 80g |
| Sat Fat | less than | 20g | 25g |
| Cholesterol | less than | 300mg | 300mg |
| Sodium | less than | 2,400mg | 2,400mg |
| Total Carbohydrate | | 300g | 375g |
| Dietary Fiber | | 25g | 30g |

**Ingredients**
GRANOLA (WHOLE GRAIN ROLLED OATS, WHOLE GRAIN ROLLED WHEAT, SUGAR, SUNFLOWER OIL, HIGH FRUCTOSE CORN SYRUP, MOLASSES, DRIED COCONUT, HONEY, SODIUM BICARBONATE, NATURAL FLAVOR, WHEY PROTEIN CONCENTRATE), SUGAR, CRISP RICE (RICE FLOUR, SUGAR, BARLEY MALT, SALT), PARTIALLY HYDROGENATED PALM KERNEL AND PALM OIL WITH GLYCERYL LACTO ESTERS OF FATTY ACIDS*, CORN SYRUP, SEMISWEET CHOCOLATE CHIPS (SUGAR, CHOCOLATE LIQUOR, COCOA BUTTER, SOY LECITHIN, VANILLA EXTRACT), HIGH FRUCTOSE CORN SYRUP, BROWN SUGAR, HYDROGENATED PALM KERNEL OIL, CORN SYRUP SOLIDS, COCOA, GLYCERIN, COCOA (PROCESSED WITH ALKALI), PARTIALLY HYDROGENATED SOYBEAN OIL*, NONFAT DRY MILK, DEMINERALIZED WHEY, LACTOSE, SORBITOL, SOY LECITHIN, SALT, NATURAL FLAVOR, BHT (A PRESERVATIVE), CITRIC ACID, WATER.
*ADDS A DIETARILY INSIGNIFICANT AMOUNT OF TRANS FAT
**CONTAINS WHEAT, COCONUT, MILK AND SOY INGREDIENTS.**
**MAY CONTAIN TRACES OF PEANUT AND OTHER TREE NUTS.**

Rating 4/10

# PEANUT BUTTERCHOCOLATE

Serving size 1 Bar (31g)
Servings Per Container 6

**Amount per serving**

| | | Calories |
|---|---|---|
| Calories 140 | | from |
| | | Fat 50 |

| | %daily value* |
|---|---|
| Total Fat 6g | 10% |
| Saturated Fat 4.5g | 21% |
| Trans Fat 0g | |
| Polyunsaturated Fat 0g | |
| Monounsaturated Fat 1g | |
| Cholesterol 0mg | 0% |
| Sodium 65mg | 3% |
| Total Carbohydrate 21g | 7% |
| Dietary Fiber 1g | 4% |
| Sugars 12g | |
| Sugar Alcohol 1g | |
| Protein 2g | |
| Iron | 2% |

Not a significant source of
Vitamin A, Vitamin C and
Calcium.
*Percent Daily Values are based
on a 2,000 calorie diet. Your daily
values may be higher or lower
depending on your calorie needs:

| | Calories | 2,000 | 2,500 |
|---|---|---|---|
| Total Fat | less than | 65g | 80g |
| Sat. Fat | less than | 20g | 25g |
| Cholesterol | less than | 300mg | 300mg |
| Sodium | less than | 2,400mg | 2,400mg |
| Total Carbohydrate | | 300g | 375g |
| Dietary Fiber | | 25g | 30g |

**Ingredients**
GRANOLA (WHOLE GRAIN ROLLED OATS, WHOLE GRAIN ROLLED WHEAT, SUGAR, SUNFLOWER OIL, HIGH FRUCTOSE CORN SYRUP, MOLASSES, DRIED COCONUT, HONEY, SODIUM BICARBONATE, NATURAL FLAVOR, WHEY PROTEIN CONCENTRATE), SUGAR, PALM KERNEL AND PALM OIL, CRISP RICE (RICE FLOUR, SUGAR, BARLEY MALT, SALT), SEMISWEET CHOCOLATE CHIPS (SUGAR, CHOCOLATE LIQUOR, COCOA BUTTER, SOY LECITHIN, VANILLA EXTRACT), CORN SYRUP, PARTIALLY DEFATTED PEANUT FLOUR, HIGH FRUCTOSE CORN SYRUP, CORN SYRUP SOLIDS, BROWN SUGAR, GLYCERIN, LACTOSE, PARTIALLY HYDROGENATED SOYBEAN OIL*, WHEY POWDER, DEXTROSE, SORBITOL, COCOA (PROCESSED WITH ALKALI), SALT, SOY LECITHIN, ARTIFICIAL FLAVOR, BHT (PRESERVATIVE), CITRIC ACID, WATER.

*ADDS A DIETARILY INSIGNIFICANT AMOUNT OF TRANS FAT

**CONTAINS WHEAT, COCONUT, MILK, SOY AND PEANUT INGREDIENTS.**
**MAY CONTAIN TRACES OF OTHER TREE NUTS.**

Rating:3.5/10 Stars

# QUAKER® BIG CHEWY SWEET & SALTY GRANOLA BARS

## CHOCOLATE & SALTED CARAMEL

Serving Size 1 bar (40 g)

Servings per Container See Table

| Amount Per Serving | | |
|---|---|---|
| **Calories** 170 | Calories from Fat 50 | |

| | %Daily Value* |
|---|---|
| **Total Fat** 6g | **9%** |
| Saturated Fat 3g | **15%** |
| Trans Fat 0g | |
| Polyunsaturated Fat 1.5g | |
| Monounsaturated Fat 1g | |
| **Cholesterol** 0mg | **0%** |
| **Sodium** 115mg | **5%** |
| **Total Carbohydrate** 29g | **10%** |
| Dietary Fiber 3g | **10%** |
| Sugars 12g | |
| Sugar Alcohol 1g | |
| **Protein** 2g | |

| | | | |
|---|---|---|---|
| Vitamin A 0% | • | Vitamin C 0% | |
| Calcium 15% | • | Iron 10% | |
| Vitamin E 0% | • | Thiamin 4% | |
| Riboflavin 2% | • | Niacin 2% | |
| Vitamin B6 2% | • | Folic Acid 4% | |
| Zinc 2% | | | |

*Percent(%) Daily Values are based on a 2,000 calorie diet. Your daily values may be higher or lower based on your calorie needs.

| | Calories | 2,000 | 2,500 |
|---|---|---|---|
| Total Fat | less than | 65g | 80g |
| Saturated Fat | less than | 20g | 25g |
| Cholesterol | less than | 300mg | 300mg |
| Sodium | less than | 2,400mg | 2,400mg |
| Total Carbohydrate | | 300g | 375g |
| Dietary Fiber | | 25g | 30g |

Calories per gram
Fat 9 • Carbohydrates 4 • Protein 4

**Ingredients**
GRANOLA (WHOLE GRAIN ROLLED OATS, BROWN SUGAR, CRISP RICE [RICE FLOUR, SUGAR, SALT, MALTED BARLEY EXTRACT], WHOLE GRAIN ROLLED WHEAT, SOYBEAN OIL, WHOLE WHEAT FLOUR, SODIUM BICARBONATE, SOY LECITHIN, CARAMEL COLOR, NONFAT DRY MILK), CORN SYRUP, SUGAR, SEMISWEET CHOCOLATE CHIPS (SUGAR, CHOCOLATE LIQUOR, COCOA BUTTER, SOY LECITHIN, VANILLA EXTRACT), OAT CEREAL (WHOLE GRAIN OAT FLOUR, WHOLE WHEAT FLOUR, BROWN SUGAR, SUGAR, MALTODEXTRIN, MALTED BARLEY EXTRACT, NATURAL FLAVOR, MOLASSES, SALT, CALCIUM CARBONATE, SODIUM BICARBONATE, SODIUM ASCORBATE, REDUCED IRON, ALPHA TOCOPHEROL ACETATE, BHT (PRESERVATIVE), NIACINAMIDE, YELLOW 5, ZINC OXIDE, YELLOW 6, THIAMIN MONONITRATE, FOLIC ACID, PYRIDOXINE HYDROCHLORIDE, VITAMIN A PALMITATE, RIBOFLAVIN), PRETZELS (ENRICHED FLOUR [WHEAT FLOUR, NIACIN, REDUCED IRON, THIAMINE MONONITRATE, RIBOFLAVIN, FOLIC ACID], CORN SYRUP, SALT, MALT SYRUP, AMMONIUM BICARBONATE, SODIUM BICARBONATE), BROWN RICE CRISPS (WHOLE GRAIN BROWN RICE FLOUR, SUGAR, MALTED BARLEY FLOUR, SALT), VEGETABLE OIL (PALM KERNEL AND PALM OIL), OLIGOFRUCTOSE, CORN SYRUP SOLIDS, SOYBEAN OIL, GLYCERIN, CALCIUM CARBONATE, REDUCED MINERAL WHEY POWDER, WATER, HONEY, NATURAL AND ARTIFICIAL FLAVOR, SALT, SOY LECITHIN, NONFAT DRY MILK, YELLOW 6 LAKE, YELLOW 5 LAKE, BHT (PRESERVATIVE), BLUE 2 LAKE, CARAMEL COLOR.

MAY CONTAIN TRACES OF PEANUTS AND TREE NUTS
CONTAINS MILK, SOY AND WHEAT INGREDIENTS.

## RATING: 4/10 STARS

## QUAKER® BIG CHEWY SWEET & SALTY GRANOLA BARS

# CARAMEL POPCORN CRUNCH

| Serving Size 1.41 OZ(40 g) | | |
|---|---|---|
| Servings per Container See Table | | |

| Amount Per Serving | | |
|---|---|---|
| Calories 170 | Calories from Fat 45 | |
| | | %Daily Value* |
| **Total Fat** 5g | | **8%** |
| Saturated Fat 2.5g | | **13%** |
| Trans Fat 0g | | |
| Polyunsaturated Fat 1.5g | | |
| Monounsaturated Fat 1g | | |
| **Cholesterol** 0mg | | **0%** |
| **Sodium** 100mg | | **4%** |
| **Total Carbohydrate** 29g | | **10%** |
| Dietary Fiber 3g | | **10%** |
| Sugars 12g | | |
| Sugar Alcohol 1g | | |
| **Protein** 2g | | |

| | | |
|---|---|---|
| Vitamin A 0% | • | Vitamin C 0% |
| Calcium 15% | • | Iron 10% |
| Vitamin E 0% | • | Thiamin 4% |
| Riboflavin 2% | • | Niacin 2% |
| Vitamin B6 2% | • | Folic Acid 4% |
| Zinc 2% | | |

* Percent(%) Daily Values are based on a 2,000 calorie diet. Your daily values may be higher or lower based on your calorie needs.

| | Calories | 2,000 | 2,500 |
|---|---|---|---|
| Total Fat | less than | 65g | 80g |
| Saturated Fat | less than | 20g | 25g |
| Cholesterol | less than | 300mg | 300mg |
| Sodium | less than | 2,400mg | 2,400mg |
| Total Carbohydrate | | 300g | 375g |
| Dietary Fiber | | 25g | 30g |

Calories per gram
Fat 9 • Carbohydrates 4 • Protein 4

**Ingredients**
GRANOLA (WHOLE GRAIN ROLLED OATS, BROWN SUGAR, CRISP RICE [RICE FLOUR, SUGAR, SALT, MALTED BARLEY EXTRACT], WHOLE GRAIN ROLLED WHEAT, SOYBEAN OIL, WHOLE WHEAT FLOUR, SODIUM BICARBONATE, SOY LECITHIN, CARAMEL COLOR, NONFAT DRY MILK), CORN SYRUP, CARAMEL CORN (CORN SYRUP, SUGAR, POPCORN, MOLASSES, SALT, SOYBEAN OIL, SOY LECITHIN), OAT CEREAL (WHOLE GRAIN OAT FLOUR, WHOLE WHEAT FLOUR, BROWN SUGAR, SUGAR, MALTODEXTRIN, MALTED BARLEY EXTRACT, NATURAL FLAVOR, MOLASSES, SALT, CALCIUM CARBONATE, SODIUM BICARBONATE, SODIUM ASCORBATE, REDUCED IRON, ALPHA TOCOPHEROL ACETATE, BHT (PRESERVATIVE), NIACINAMIDE, YELLOW 5, ZINC OXIDE, YELLOW 6, THIAMIN MONONITRATE, FOLIC ACID, PYRIDOXINE HYDROCHLORIDE, VITAMIN A PALMITATE, RIBOFLAVIN), SUGAR, PRETZELS (ENRICHED FLOUR [WHEAT FLOUR, NIACIN, REDUCED IRON, THIAMIN MONONITRATE, RIBOFLAVIN, FOLIC ACID], CORN SYRUP, SALT, MALT SYRUP, AMMONIUM BICARBONATE, SODIUM BICARBONATE), VEGETABLE OIL (PALM KERNEL AND PALM OIL), OLIGOFRUCTOSE, CORN SYRUP SOLIDS, SOYBEAN OIL, BROWN RICE CRISP (WHOLE GRAIN BROWN RICE FLOUR, SUGAR, MALTED BARLEY FLOUR, SALT), GLYCERIN, COCOA (PROCESSED WITH ALKALI), NATURAL AND ARTIFICIAL FLAVOR, COCOA POWDER, CALCIUM CARBONATE, DRY WHEY, NONFAT DRY MILK, WATER, HONEY, LACTOSE, SOY LECITHIN, SALT, VANILLA EXTRACT, BHT (PRESERVATIVE), CARAMEL COLOR.

**CONTAINS WHEAT, MILK AND SOY INGREDIENTS.**
**MAY CONTAIN TRACES OF PEANUT AND TREE NUTS**

## Rating: 4.5/10 Stars

## QUAKER® BIG CHEWY® GRANOLA BARS

## CHOCOLATE CHIP WITH DARK CHOCOLATY DRIZZLE

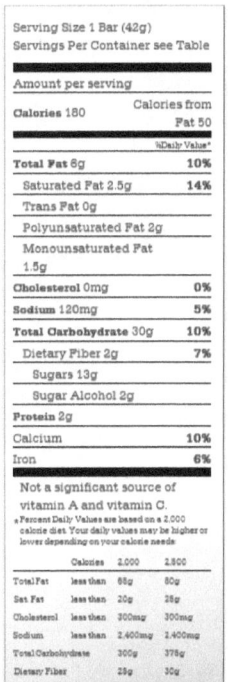

Serving Size 1 Bar (42g)
Servings Per Container see Table

Amount per serving

Calories 180 — Calories from Fat 50

| | %Daily Value* |
|---|---|
| Total Fat 6g | 10% |
| Saturated Fat 2.5g | 14% |
| Trans Fat 0g | |
| Polyunsaturated Fat 2g | |
| Monounsaturated Fat 1.5g | |
| Cholesterol 0mg | 0% |
| Sodium 120mg | 5% |
| Total Carbohydrate 30g | 10% |
| Dietary Fiber 2g | 7% |
| Sugars 13g | |
| Sugar Alcohol 2g | |
| Protein 2g | |
| Calcium | 10% |
| Iron | 6% |

Not a significant source of vitamin A and vitamin C.

* Percent Daily Values are based on a 2,000 calorie diet. Your daily values may be higher or lower depending on your calorie needs

| | Calories | 2,000 | 2,500 |
|---|---|---|---|
| Total Fat | less than | 65g | 80g |
| Sat Fat | less than | 20g | 25g |
| Cholesterol | less than | 300mg | 300mg |
| Sodium | less than | 2,400mg | 2,400mg |
| Total Carbohydrate | | 300g | 375g |
| Dietary Fiber | | 25g | 30g |

**Ingredients**
Granola (Wheat Grain Rolled Oats, Brown Sugar, Crisp Rice [Rice Flour, Sugar, Salt, Malted Barley Extract], Whole Grain Rolled Wheat, Soybean Oil, Dried Coconut, Whole Wheat Flour, Sodium Bicarbonate, Soy Lecithin, Caramel Color, Nonfat Dry Milk). Semisweet Chocolate Chips (Sugar, Chocolate Liquor, Cocoa Butter, Soy Lecithin, Vanilla Extract). Corn Syrup, Sugar, Brown Rice Crisp (Whole Grain Brown Rice, Sugar, Malted Barley Flour, Salt). Invert Sugar, Cron Syrup Solids, Glycerin, Soybean Oil, Vegetable Oil( Palm Oil,Palm Kernel Oil). Contains 2% or Less of Sorbitol, Calcium Carbonate, Cocoa Powder (Processed with Alkali), Salt, Cocoa Powder, Water, Whey, NonFat Dry Milk, Lactose, Soy Lecithin, Molasses, Natural and Artificial Flavor, Vanilla Extract, BHT (Preservative). Citric Acid.

CONTAINS WHEAT, COCONUT, SOY AND MILK INGREDIENTS.
MAY CONTAIN TRACES OF PEANUT AND OTEHR TREE NUTS.
31407-1

Rating: 4.5 /10 Stars

# QUAKER® BIG CHEWY® GRANOLA BARS

## PEANUT BUTTERCHOCOLATE CHIP

| Serving Size 1 Bar (42g) | |
|---|---|
| Servings Per Container 5 | |

| Amount per serving | |
|---|---|
| **Calories** 180 | Calories from Fat 50 |

| | %Daily Value* |
|---|---|
| **Total Fat** 6g | **9%** |
| Saturated Fat 2.5g | **12%** |
| Trans Fat 0g | |
| Polyunsaturated Fat 1g | |
| Monounsaturated Fat 2g | |
| **Cholesterol** 0mg | **0%** |
| **Sodium** 160mg | **7%** |
| **Total Carbohydrate** 30g | **10%** |
| Dietary Fiber 2g | **7%** |
| Sugars 13g | |
| Sugar Alcohol 2g | |
| **Protein** 3g | |
| Calcium | **15%** |
| Iron | **6%** |

Not a significant source of vitamin A and vitamin C.

* Percent Daily Values are based on a 2,000 calorie diet. Your daily values may be higher or lower depending on your calorie needs:

| | Calories | 2,000 | 2,500 |
|---|---|---|---|
| Total Fat | less than | 65g | 80g |
| Sat. Fat | less than | 20g | 25g |
| Cholesterol | less than | 300mg | 300mg |
| Sodium | less than | 2,400mg | 2,400mg |
| Total Carbohydrate | | 300g | 375g |
| Dietary Fiber | | 25g | 30g |

**Ingredients**
GRANOLA (WHOLE GRAIN ROLLED OATS, BROWN SUGAR, CRISP RICE [RICE FLOUR, SUGAR, SALT, MALTED BARLEY EXTRACT], WHOLE GRAIN ROLLED WHEAT, SOYBEAN OIL, WHOLE WHEAT FLOUR, SODIUM BICARBONATE, SOY LECITHIN, CARAMEL COLOR, NONFAT DRY MILK), CORN SYRUP, BROWN RICE CRISP (WHOLE GRAIN BROWN RICE, SUGAR, MALTED BARLEY FLOUR, SALT), PEANUT BUTTER SPREAD (PEANUTS, SUGAR, PALM OIL, SALT), SEMISWEET CHOCOLATE CHIPS (SUGAR, CHOCOLATE LIQUOR, COCOA BUTTER, SOY LECITHIN, VANILLA EXTRACT), INVERT SUGAR, PEANUT FLAVORED CHIPS (SUGAR, PALM KERNEL AND PALM OIL, PARTIALLY DEFATTED PEANUT FLOUR, LACTOSE, WHEY, DEXTROSE, CORN SYRUP SOLIDS, SOY LECITHIN, SALT, VANILLIN [ARTIFICIAL FLAVOR]), CORN SYRUP SOLIDS, SUGAR, GLYCERIN.CONTAINS 2% OR LESS OF PALM KERNEL AND PALM OIL, CALCIUM CARBONATE, SORBITOL, PARTIALLY DEFATTED PEANUT FLOUR, SALT, LACTOSE, WHEY, DEXTROSE, WATER, SOY LECITHIN, NATURAL AND ARTIFICIAL FLAVOR, BHT (PRESERVATIVE), CITRIC ACID.

CONTAINS WHEAT, SOY, PEANUT AND MILK INGREDIENTS.
MAY CONTAIN TRACES OF TREE NUTS.
31685-1

Rating: 5/10 Stars

The big chewy are basically larger versions of the regular chewy bars which is why they have more calories. For a review of these bars just refer back to the chewy bars.

## *QUAKER® 25% LESS SUGAR CHEWY GRANOLA BARS*

## CHOCOLATE CHIP

| Serving size 1 Bar (24g) | |
|---|---|
| **Amount per serving** | |
| | Calories |
| Calories 100 | from Fat 30 |
| | %daily value |
| Total Fat 3.5g | 6% |
| Saturated Fat 1g | 5% |
| Trans Fat 0g | |
| Sodium 75mg | 3% |
| Total Carbohydrate 17g | 6% |
| Dietary Fiber 3g | 11% |
| Sugars 5g | |
| Protein 1g | |
| Calcium 10% • Iron 2% | |

Not a significant source of Cholesterol, Vitamin A, Vitamin C.

*Percent Daily Values are based on a 2,000 calorie diet. Your daily values may be higher or lower depending on your calorie needs.

| | Calories | 2,000 | 2,500 |
|---|---|---|---|
| Total Fat | less than | 65g | 80g |
| Sat Fat | less than | 20g | 25g |
| Cholesterol | less than | 300mg | 300mg |
| Sodium | less than | 2,400mg | 2,400mg |
| Total Carbohydrate | | 300g | 375g |
| Dietary Fiber | | 25g | 30g |

**Ingredients**
GRANOLA (WHOLE GRAIN ROLLED OATS, BROWN SUGAR, CRISP RICE [RICE FLOUR, SUGAR, SALT, MALTED BARLEY EXTRACT], WHOLE GRAIN ROLLED WHEAT, SOYBEAN OIL, DRIED COCONUT, WHOLE WHEAT FLOUR, SODIUM BICARBONATE, SOY LECITHIN, CARAMEL COLOR, NONFAT DRY MILK), CORN SYRUP, SEMISWEET CHOCOLATE CHIPS (SUGAR, CHOCOLATE LIQUOR, COCOA BUTTER, SOY LECITHIN, VANILLA EXTRACT), BROWN RICE CRISP (WHOLE GRAIN BROWN RICE, SUGAR, MALTED BARLEY FLOUR, SALT), SUNFLOWER OIL, OLIGOFRUCTOSE, POLYDEXTROSE, CORN SYRUP SOLIDS, GLYCERIN. CONTAINS 2% OR LESS OF WATER, CALCIUM CARBONATE, INVERT SUGAR, SALT, MOLASSES, DIACETYL TARTARIC ACID ESTER OF MONO-DIGLYCERIDES, SUCRALOSE, NATURAL AND ARTIFICIAL FLAVOR, BHT (PRESERVATIVE), CITRIC ACID.

**Kosher Status**: Kosher Dairy

*ADDS A DIETARILY INSIGNIFICANT AMOUNT OF TRANS FAT

**CONTAINS WHEAT, SOY AND MILK INGREDIENTS.**
**MAY CONTAIN TRACES OF PEANUT AND OTHER TREE NUTS.**

**Rating: 4.5 /10 Stars**

# QUAKER® 25% LESS SUGAR CHEWY GRANOLA BARS

## COOKIES AND CREAM

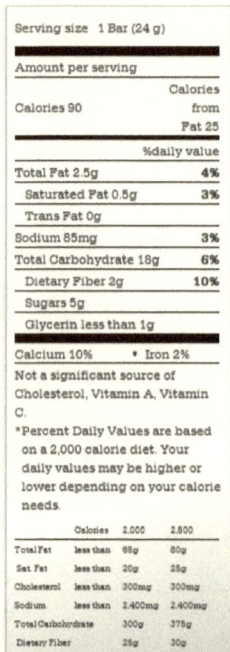

| | |
|---|---|
| Serving size 1 Bar (24 g) | |

| Amount per serving | |
|---|---|
| | Calories |
| Calories 90 | from |
| | Fat 25 |

| | %daily value |
|---|---|
| Total Fat 2.5g | 4% |
| Saturated Fat 0.5g | 3% |
| Trans Fat 0g | |
| Sodium 85mg | 3% |
| Total Carbohydrate 18g | 6% |
| Dietary Fiber 2g | 10% |
| Sugars 5g | |
| Glycerin less than 1g | |

| Calcium 10% | • Iron 2% |
|---|---|

Not a significant source of Cholesterol, Vitamin A, Vitamin C.

*Percent Daily Values are based on a 2,000 calorie diet. Your daily values may be higher or lower depending on your calorie needs.

| | Calories | 2,000 | 2,500 |
|---|---|---|---|
| Total Fat | less than | 65g | 80g |
| Sat Fat | less than | 20g | 25g |
| Cholesterol | less than | 300mg | 300mg |
| Sodium | less than | 2,400mg | 2,400mg |
| Total Carbohydrate | | 300g | 375g |
| Dietary Fiber | | 25g | 30g |

**Ingredients**
GRANOLA (WHOLE GRAIN ROLLED OATS, BROWN SUGAR, CRISP RICE [RICE FLOUR, SUGAR, SALT, MALTED BARLEY EXTRACT], WHOLE GRAIN ROLLED WHEAT, SOYBEAN OIL, WHOLE WHEAT FLOUR, SODIUM BICARBONATE, SOY LECITHIN, CARAMEL COLOR, NONFAT DRY MILK), BROWN RICE CRISP (WHOLE GRAIN BROWN RICE, SUGAR, MALTED BARLEY FLOUR, SALT), CORN SYRUP, CHOCOLATE COOKIE PIECES (ENRICHED FLOUR [WHEAT FLOUR, NIACIN, REDUCED IRON, THIAMIN MONONITRATE, RIBOFLAVIN, FOLIC ACID], SUGAR, SOYBEAN AND/OR PALM OILS, CARAMEL COLOR, COCOA PROCESSED WITH ALKALI, CORN FLOUR, SALT, DEXTROSE, SODIUM BICARBONATE, SOY LECITHIN), CONFECTIONERY CHIPS (SUGAR, PALM KERNEL OIL, NONFAT DRY MILK, PALM OIL, ARTIFICIAL COLOR, SOY LECITHIN), CORN SYRUP SOLIDS, OLIGOFRUCTOSE, POLYDEXTROSE, SUNFLOWER OIL, GLYCERIN, WATER. CONTAINS 2% OR LESS OF CALCIUM CARBONATE, INVERT SUGAR, SALT, FRUCTOSE, SOY LECITHIN, MOLASSES, NATURAL AND ARTIFICIAL FLAVOR, SUCRALOSE, BHT (PRESERVATIVE), CITRIC ACID.

**Kosher Status:** Kosher Dairy

*ONE OF THE B VITAMINS
**ADDS A DIETARILY INSIGNIFICANT AMOUNT OF TRANS FAT

**CONTAINS WHEAT, SOY AND MILK INGREDIENTS.
MAY CONTAIN TRACES OF PEANUT AND TREE NUTS.**

Rating: 6/10 Stars

# QUAKER® 25% LESS SUGAR CHEWY GRANOLA BARS

## PEANUT BUTTER CHOCOLATE CHIP

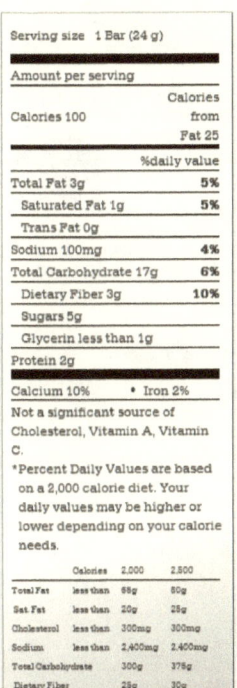

| Serving size 1 Bar (24 g) | | |
|---|---|---|
| **Amount per serving** | | |
| | | Calories |
| Calories 100 | | from Fat 25 |
| | | %daily value |
| Total Fat 3g | | 5% |
| Saturated Fat 1g | | 5% |
| Trans Fat 0g | | |
| Sodium 100mg | | 4% |
| Total Carbohydrate 17g | | 6% |
| Dietary Fiber 3g | | 10% |
| Sugars 5g | | |
| Glycerin less than 1g | | |
| Protein 2g | | |
| Calcium 10% • Iron 2% | | |

Not a significant source of Cholesterol, Vitamin A, Vitamin C.

*Percent Daily Values are based on a 2,000 calorie diet. Your daily values may be higher or lower depending on your calorie needs.

| | Calories | 2,000 | 2,500 |
|---|---|---|---|
| Total Fat | less than | 65g | 80g |
| Sat Fat | less than | 20g | 25g |
| Cholesterol | less than | 300mg | 300mg |
| Sodium | less than | 2,400mg | 2,400mg |
| Total Carbohydrate | | 300g | 375g |
| Dietary Fiber | | 25g | 30g |

**Ingredients**

INGREDIENTS: GRANOLA (WHOLE GRAIN ROLLED OATS, BROWN SUGAR, CRISP RICE [RICE FLOUR, SUGAR, SALT, MALTED BARLEY EXTRACT], WHOLE GRAIN ROLLED WHEAT, SOYBEAN OIL, WHOLE WHEAT FLOUR, SODIUM BICARBONATE, SOY LECITHIN, CARAMEL COLOR, NONFAT DRY MILK), BROWN RICE CRISP (WHOLE GRAIN BROWN RICE, SUGAR, MALTED BARLEY FLOUR, SALT), PEANUT BUTTER SPREAD (PEANUTS, SUGAR, PALM OIL, SALT), CORN SYRUP, SEMISWEET CHOCOLATE CHIPS (SUGAR, CHOCOLATE LIQUOR, COCOA BUTTER, SOY LECITHIN, VANILLA EXTRACT), PEANUT FLAVORED CHIPS (SUGAR, PALM KERNEL AND PALM OIL, PARTIALLY DEFATTED PEANUT FLOUR, LACTOSE, DRY WHEY, DEXTROSE, CORN SYRUP SOLIDS, SOY LECITHIN, SALT, VANILLIN [ARTIFICIAL FLAVOR]), OLIGOFRUCTOSE, POLYDEXTROSE, GLYCERIN, WATER.

CONTAINS 2% OR LESS OF CORN SYRUP SOLIDS, INVERT SUGAR, CALCIUM CARBONATE, SALT, SOYBEAN OIL, NATURAL AND ARTIFICIAL FLAVOR, SUCRALOSE, BHT (PRESERVATIVE), CITRIC ACID.

**CONTAINS WHEAT, PEANUT, SOY AND MILK INGREDIENTS.**

**MAY CONTAIN TRACES OF TREE NUTS.**

I am very vigilant when I see signs of reduced sugar or reduced calorie bars. The reason for this is that usually, When they reduce sugars, they substitute with starch or possibly a sugar substitute that can be equally harmful.
Rating: 5.5/10 Stars

# QUAKER® CHEWY 90 CALORIE GRANOLA BARS

## CHOCOLATE CHUNK

Serving size 1 bar (24g)

| Amount per serving | |
|---|---|
| | Calories |
| Calories 90 | from |
| | Fat 20 |

| | %daily value |
|---|---|
| Total Fat 2g | **3%** |
| Saturated Fat 0.5g | **2%** |
| Trans Fat 0g | |
| Cholesterol 0mg | **0%** |
| Sodium 80mg | **3%** |
| Total Carbohydrate 19g | **6%** |
| Dietary Fiber 1g | **4%** |
| Sugars 7g | |
| Protein 1g | |

Calcium 8%  •  Iron 2%

Not a significant source of Cholesterol, Vitamin A, Vitamin C.

*Percent Daily Values are based on a 2,000 calorie diet. Your daily values may be higher or lower depending on your calorie needs.

| | Calories | 2,000 | 2,500 |
|---|---|---|---|
| Total Fat | less than | 65g | 80g |
| Sat Fat | less than | 20g | 25g |
| Cholesterol | less than | 300mg | 300mg |
| Sodium | less than | 2,400mg | 2,400mg |
| Total Carbohydrate | | 300g | 375g |
| Dietary Fiber | | 25g | 30g |

**Ingredients**
GRANOLA (WHOLE GRAIN ROLLED OATS, BROWN SUGAR, CRISP RICE [RICE FLOUR, SUGAR, SALT, MALTED BARLEY EXTRACT], WHOLE GRAIN ROLLED WHEAT, SOYBEAN OIL, WHOLE WHEAT FLOUR, SODIUM BICARBONATE, SOY LECITHIN, CARAMEL COLOR, NONFAT DRY MILK), CORN SYRUP, BROWN RICE CRISP (WHOLE GRAIN BROWN RICE, SUGAR, MALTED BARLEY FLOUR, SALT), SEMISWEET CHOCOLATE CHUNKS (SUGAR, CHOCOLATE LIQUOR, COCOA BUTTER, SOY LECITHIN, VANILLIN [AN ARTIFICIAL FLAVOR]), SUGAR, CORN SYRUP SOLIDS, GLYCERIN, INVERT SUGAR.CONTAINS 2% OR LESS OF SOYBEAN OIL, SORBITOL, FRUCTOSE, CALCIUM CARBONATE, SALT, SOY LECITHIN, MOLASSES, NATURAL AND ARTIFICIAL FLAVOR, WATER, CREAMED COCONUT, BHT (PRESERVATIVE), CITRIC ACID.

**Kosher Status**: Kosher Dairy

**CONTAINS WHEAT, SOY, MILK AND COCONUT INGREDIENTS.
MAY CONTAIN TRACES OF PEANUTS AND OTHER TREE NUTS.**

## Rating: 6/10 Stars

# QUAKER® CHEWY 90 CALORIE GRANOLA BARS

## OATMEAL RAISIN

| Nutrition Facts | |
|---|---|
| Serving size 1 bar (24g) | |

| Amount per serving | |
|---|---|
| | Calories |
| Calories 90 | from |
| | Fat 15 |

| | %daily value |
|---|---|
| Total Fat 1.5g | 3% |
| Saturated Fat 0g | 0% |
| Trans Fat 0g | |
| Cholesterol 0mg | 0% |
| Sodium 80mg | 3% |
| Total Carbohydrate 19g | 6% |
| Dietary Fiber 1g | 4% |
| Sugars 7g | |
| Protein 1g | |

| Calcium 8% | • Iron 2% |
|---|---|

Not a significant source of Cholesterol, Vitamin A, Vitamin C.

*Percent Daily Values are based on a 2,000 calorie diet. Your daily values may be higher or lower depending on your calorie needs.

| | Calories | 2,000 | 2,500 |
|---|---|---|---|
| Total Fat | less than | 65g | 80g |
| Sat Fat | less than | 20g | 25g |
| Cholesterol | less than | 300mg | 300mg |
| Sodium | less than | 2,400mg | 2,400mg |
| Total Carbohydrate | | 300g | 375g |
| Dietary Fiber | | 25g | 30g |

**Ingredients**

GRANOLA (WHOLE GRAIN ROLLED OATS, BROWN SUGAR, CRISP RICE [RICE FLOUR, SUGAR, SALT, MALTED BARLEY EXTRACT], WHOLE GRAIN ROLLED WHEAT, SOYBEAN OIL, WHOLE WHEAT FLOUR, SODIUM BICARBONATE, SOY LECITHIN, CARAMEL COLOR, NONFAT DRY MILK), CORN SYRUP, BROWN RICE CRISP (WHOLE GRAIN BROWN RICE, SUGAR, MALTED BARLEY FLOUR, SALT), RAISINS, OATMEAL COOKIE PIECES (SUGAR, ENRICHED FLOUR [WHEAT FLOUR, NIACIN*, REDUCED IRON, THIAMIN MONONITRATE*, RIBOFLAVIN*, FOLIC ACID*], OATS, SOYBEAN AND/OR PALM OILS, WHOLE WHEAT FLOUR, CINNAMON, SALT, SODIUM BICARBONATE), SUGAR, CORN SYRUP SOLIDS, GLYCERIN, INVERT SUGAR, SOYBEAN OIL. CONTAINS 2% OR LESS OF SORBITOL, CALCIUM CARBONATE, FRUCTOSE, SALT, MOLASSES, SOY LECITHIN, NATURAL AND ARTIFICIAL FLAVOR, CINNAMON, CREAMED COCONUT, BHT (PRESERVATIVE), WATER, CITRIC ACID. *ONE OF THE B VITAMINS

**CONTAINS WHEAT, SOY, MILK AND COCONUT INGREDIENTS.**

**MAY CONTAIN TRACES OF PEANUT AND OTHER TREE NUTS.**

Rating: 6.3/10 Stars

# QUAKER® CHEWY 90 CALORIE GRANOLA BARS

## PEANUT BUTTER

| Serving size 1 Bar (24g) | |
|---|---|
| **Amount per serving** | |
| | Calories |
| Calories 90 | from |
| | Fat 20 |
| | %daily value |
| Total Fat 2g | **3%** |
| Saturated Fat 0g | **0%** |
| Trans Fat 0g | |
| Sodium 120mg | **5%** |
| Total Carbohydrate 18g | **6%** |
| Dietary Fiber 1g | **4%** |
| Sugars 7g | |
| Protein 2g | |
| Calcium 10% • Iron 2% | |

Not a significant source of Cholesterol, Vitamin A, Vitamin C.

*Percent Daily Values are based on a 2,000 calorie diet. Your daily values may be higher or lower depending on your calorie needs.

| | Calories | 2,000 | 2,500 |
|---|---|---|---|
| Total Fat | less than | 65g | 80g |
| Sat. Fat | less than | 20g | 25g |
| Cholesterol | less than | 300mg | 300mg |
| Sodium | less than | 2,400mg | 2,400mg |
| Total Carbohydrate | | 300g | 375g |
| Dietary Fiber | | 25g | 30g |

**Ingredients**
GRANOLA (WHOLE GRAIN ROLLED OATS, BROWN SUGAR, CRISP RICE [RICE FLOUR, SUGAR, SALT, MALTED BARLEY EXTRACT], WHOLE GRAIN ROLLED WHEAT, SOYBEAN OIL, WHOLE WHEAT FLOUR, SODIUM BICARBONATE, SOY LECITHIN, CARAMEL COLOR, NONFAT DRY MILK), BROWN RICE CRISP (WHOLE GRAIN BROWN RICE, SUGAR, MALTED BARLEY FLOUR, SALT), CORN SYRUP, INVERT SUGAR, PEANUT BUTTER SPREAD (PEANUTS, SUGAR, PALM OIL, SALT), SUGAR, GLYCERIN, CORN SYRUP SOLIDS.CONTAINS 2% OR LESS OF SORBITOL, CALCIUM CARBONATE, SALT, NATURAL AND ARTIFICIAL FLAVOR, BHT (PRESERVATIVE), WATER, CITRIC ACID.

**CONTAINS WHEAT, PEANUT, SOY AND MILK INGREDIENTS.**

**MAY CONTAIN TRACES OF TREE NUTS.**

Rating: 4/10 Stars

# QUAKER® CHEWY 90 CALORIE GRANOLA BARS

## Smores

**Serving size** 1 bar (24g)

| Amount per serving | |
|---|---|
| | Calories |
| Calories 90 | from Fat 20 |
| | %daily value |
| Total Fat 2g | 3% |
| Saturated Fat 0.5g | 2% |
| Trans Fat 0g | |
| Cholesterol 0mg | 0% |
| Sodium 75mg | 3% |
| Total Carbohydrate 19g | 6% |
| Dietary Fiber 1g | 3% |
| Sugars 8g | |
| Protein 1g | |
| Calcium 8% • Iron 2% | |

Not a significant source of Cholesterol, Vitamin A, Vitamin C.
*Percent Daily Values are based on a 2,000 calorie diet. Your daily values may be higher or lower depending on your calorie needs.

| | Calories | 2,000 | 2,500 |
|---|---|---|---|
| Total Fat | less than | 65g | 80g |
| Sat Fat | less than | 20g | 25g |
| Cholesterol | less than | 300mg | 300mg |
| Sodium | less than | 2,400mg | 2,400mg |
| Total Carbohydrate | | 300g | 375g |
| Dietary Fiber | | 25g | 30g |

**Ingredients**
GRANOLA (WHOLE GRAINROLLED OATS, BROWN SUGAR, CRISP RICE [RICE FLOUR, SUGAR, SALT, MALTEDBARLEY EXTRACT], WHOLE GRAIN ROLLED WHEAT, SOYBEAN OIL, WHOLE WHEATFLOUR, SODIUM BICARBONATE, SOY LECITHIN, CARAMEL COLOR, NONFAT DRYMILK), CORN SYRUP, BROWN RICE CRISP (WHOLE GRAIN BROWN RICE, SUGAR,MALTED BARLEY FLOUR, SALT), SEMISWEET CHOCOLATE CHIPS (SUGAR,CHOCOLATE LIQUOR, COCOA BUTTER, SOY LECITHIN, VANILLA EXTRACT),SUGAR, DEHYDRATED MARSHMALLOWS (SUGAR, CORN SYRUP, MODIFIED FOODSTARCH, GELATIN, NATURAL AND ARTIFICIAL FLAVOR, SODIUMHEXAMETAPHOSPHATE, BLUE 1), CORN SYRUP SOLIDS, INVERT SUGAR,GLYCERIN, GRAHAM COOKIE PIECES (SUGAR, WHOLE WHEAT FLOUR, WHEATFLOUR, CANOLA OIL, HONEY POWDER, SODIUM BICARBONATE, SALT, SOYLECITHIN, NATURAL FLAVOR).
CONTAINS 2% OR LESS OF SOYBEAN OIL,SORBITOL, CALCIUM CARBONATE, SALT, WATER, MOLASSES, SOY LECITHIN,NATURAL AND ARTIFICIAL FLAVOR, CREAMED COCONUT, BHT (PRESERVATIVE),CITRIC ACID.

**CONTAINS WHEAT, SOY, MILK ANDCOCONUT INGREDIENTS.
MAY CONTAIN TRACES OF PEANUT ANDOTHER TREE NUTS.**

## Rating:6/10 Stars

This is a very low calorie bar. I like that this bar has granola as the first ingredient. Also it doesn't have any high fructose corn syrup (Quaker stopped using it). It is obviously a low calorie bar (only 90 calories) and is low calorie as well. It does have a bit of sodium and not a lot of fiber compared to its sugar content.

# Fiber One

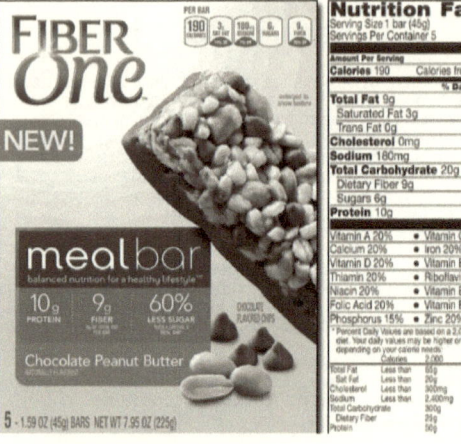

Rating 8/10 Stars
big serving size, a little high in fat, low in carbs, high in protein
Great fiber!

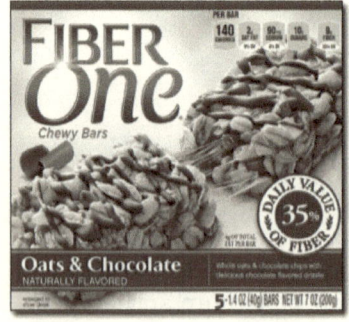
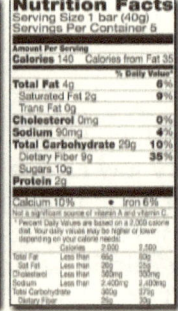

Rating: 6/10 Stars
Big serving size, high fiber, high carbs, low fat, low sodium, low protein.

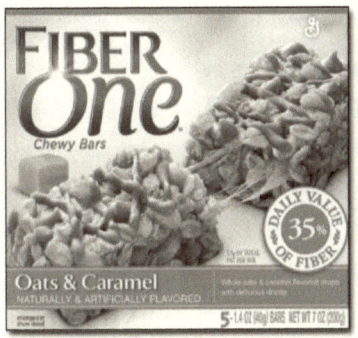 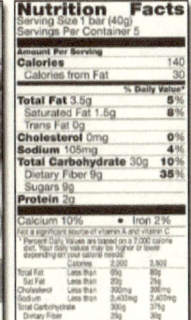

**Nutrition Facts**
Serving Size 1 bar (40g)
Servings Per Container 5

Amount Per Serving

Calories 140     Calories from Fat 30

| | % Daily Value* |
|---|---|
| **Total Fat** 3.5g | **5%** |
| Saturated Fat 1.5g | **8%** |
| Trans Fat 0g | |
| **Cholesterol** 0mg | **0%** |
| **Sodium** 105mg | **4%** |
| **Total Carbohydrate** 30g | **10%** |
| Dietary Fiber 9g | **35%** |
| Sugars 9g | |
| **Protein** 2g | |

Calcium 10%   •   Iron 2%

Ingredients: Chicory Root Extract, Whole Grain Oats, Caramel Flavored Drops (sugar, fractionated palm kernel and palm oil, reduced minerals whey, nonfat milk, dextrose, salt, soy lecithin, natural and artificial flavor, color yellows 5 & 6 lake, blue 2 lake). Rice Flour, Barley Flakes, High Maltose Corn Syrup, Sugar, Vegetable Oil (canola, fractionated palm kernel, soybean), Honey, Maltodextrin, Glycerin, Tricalcium Phosphate, Soy Lecithin, Salt, Fructose, Malt Extract, Color (yellows 6 & 5 lake, blue 2 lake and other color added), Reduced Minerals Whey, Baking Soda, Natural and Artificial Flavor, Nonfat Milk, Mixed Tocopherols and BHA Added to Retain Freshness.

CONTAINS MILK, SOY; MAY CONTAIN PEANUT, ALMOND, SUNFLOWER AND WHEAT INGREDIENTS.

DIST. BY GENERAL MILLS SALES, INC., MINNEAPOLIS, MN 55440 USA

© 2012 General Mills 3971508101

## Rating: 5.5/10 Stars

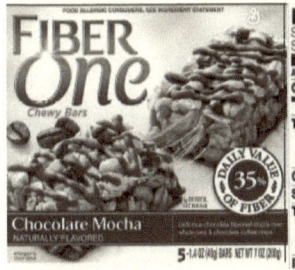

**Nutrition Facts**
Serving Size 1 bar (40g)
Servings Per Container 5

Amount Per Serving

Calories 140     Calories from Fat 40

| | % Daily Value* |
|---|---|
| **Total Fat** 4g | **6%** |
| Saturated Fat 2g | **9%** |
| Trans Fat 0g | |
| **Cholesterol** 0mg | **0%** |
| **Sodium** 95mg | **4%** |
| **Total Carbohydrate** 29g | **10%** |
| Dietary Fiber 9g | **35%** |
| Sugars 10g | |
| **Protein** 2g | |

Calcium 10%   •   Iron 2%

CLOSE **X**

Ingredients: Chicory Root Extract, Sweet Chocolate Chips with Coffee (sugar, chocolate liquor, coffee, cocoa butter, milk fat, soy lecithin, vanillin), Whole Grain Oats, Rice Flour, Barley Flakes, High Maltose Corn Syrup, Sugar, Glycerin, Honey, Canola Oil, Maltodextrin, Palm Kernel Oil, Tricalcium Phosphate, Soy Lecithin, Salt, Nonfat Milk, Fructose, Malt Extract, Cocoa Processed with Alkali, Caramel Color, Natural Flavor, Baking Soda. Mixed Tocopherols Added to Retain Freshness.

CONTAINS SOY, MILK; MAY CONTAIN WHEAT, PEANUT, ALMOND AND SUNFLOWER INGREDIENTS.

DIST. BY GENERAL MILLS SALES, INC., MINNEAPOLIS, MN 55440 USA

© 2011 General Mills 3999809105

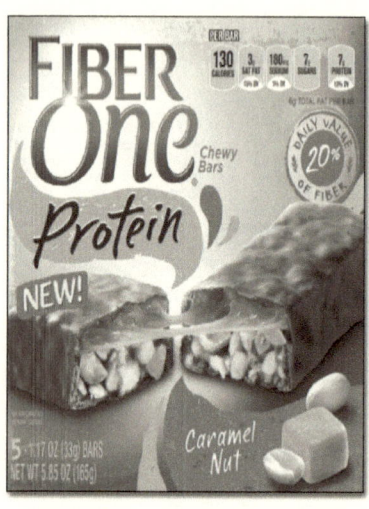

Higer protein, low carb, higher fat

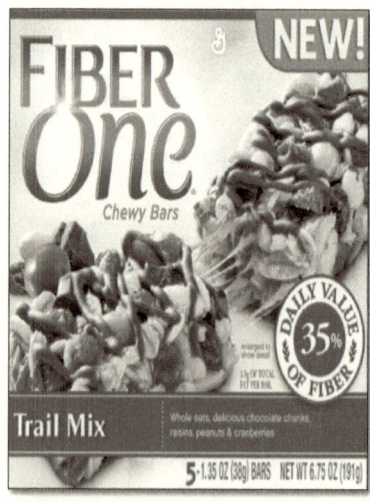

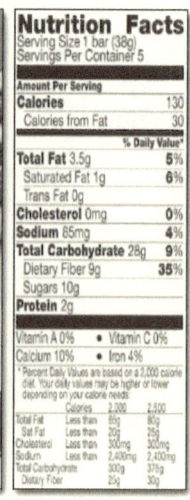

high fiber, high carb

Gerneral Rating: High fiber, medium carb, high protein, very high fat, medium valorize, not very wholesome

Rating: 3.5 Stars

## Winner Fiber One meal bar

### Why: low in fat, high in protein and low in carbs

# Chips

According to a traditional story, the original potato chip recipe was created in <u>Saratoga Springs, New York</u>. Most say the event happened on 24 August 1853 and credit <u>George Crum</u>, a half black, half <u>Native American</u> cook[2] at Moon's Lake House for the invention. The potatoe chip was invented when an unhappy customer frustrated Mr. Crum by sending his fried potatoes back, complaining that they were too thick.[3] Frustrated, he sliced the potatoes razor thin, fried them until crisp and seasoned them with extra salt. To Crum's surprise, the customer loved them.[4] They soon became called "Saratoga Chips",[5] a name that persisted into at least the mid-20th century. Chips are tasty but also, have a high fat and starch content and too many is not healthy. For this reason they should be enjoyed if daily, in a limited amount.

## Cheetos cheese puff

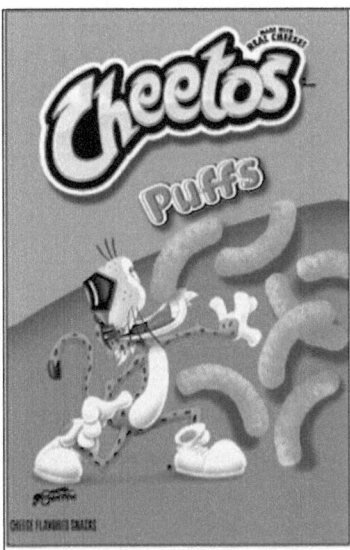

**Nutrition Facts**
Serving Size 1 oz (28g/About 13 pieces)

**Amount Per Serving**

| Calories 150 | Calories from Fat 90 |
|---|---|
| | **% Daily Value\*** |

| | % Daily Value |
|---|---|
| **Total Fat** 10g | **15%** |
| Saturated Fat 1.5g | **8%** |
| Trans Fat 0g | |
| **Cholesterol** 0mg | **0%** |
| **Sodium** 300mg | **13%** |
| **Total Carbohydrate** 13g | **4%** |
| Dietary Fiber less than 1g | **2%** |
| Sugars 1g | |
| **Protein** 2g | |

| | | |
|---|---|---|
| Vitamin A 0% | • | Vitamin C 0% |
| Calcium 2% | • | Iron 2% |
| Thiamin 8% | • | Riboflavin 4% |
| Niacin 4% | • | Vitamin B6 2% |

\* Percent Daily Values are based on a 2,000 calorie diet. Your daily values may be higher or lower depending on your calorie needs:

| | Calories: | 2,000 | 2,500 |
|---|---|---|---|
| Total Fat | Less than | 65g | 80g |
| Sat Fat | Less than | 20g | 25g |
| Cholesterol | Less than | 300mg | 300mg |
| Sodium | Less than | 2,400mg | 2,400mg |
| Total Carbohydrate | | 300g | 375g |
| Dietary Fiber | | 25g | 30g |

Calories per gram:
Fat 9 • Carbohydrate 4 • Protein 4

**Ingredients:** Enriched Corn Meal (Corn Meal, Ferrous Sulfate, Niacin, Thiamin Mononitrate, Riboflavin, and Folic Acid), Vegetable Oil (Corn, Canola, and/or Sunflower Oil), Cheese Seasoning (Whey, Cheddar Cheese [Milk, Cheese Cultures, Salt, Enzymes], Canola Oil, Maltodextrin [Made From Corn], Salt, Whey Protein Concentrate, Monosodium Glutamate, Natural and Artificial Flavors, Lactic Acid, Citric Acid, Artificial Color [Yellow 6]), and Salt.
**CONTAINS MILK INGREDIENTS.**

Rating: 3.5 /10 Stars

# Lays Barbecue

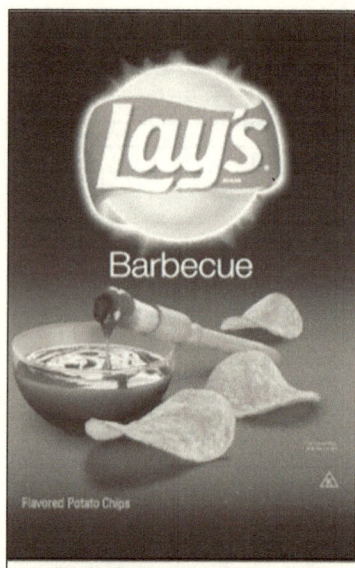

**Nutrition Facts**
Serving Size 1 oz (28g/About 15 chips)

**Amount Per Serving**

**Calories** 160     Calories from Fat 90

| | % Daily Value* |
|---|---|
| **Total Fat** 10g | **15%** |
| Saturated Fat 1.5g | **7%** |
| Trans Fat 0g | |
| **Cholesterol** 0mg | **0%** |
| **Sodium** 150mg | **6%** |
| **Potassium** 320mg | **9%** |
| **Total Carbohydrate** 15g | **5%** |
| Dietary Fiber 1g | **5%** |
| Sugars 2g | |
| **Protein** 2g | |

| Vitamin A 0% | • | Vitamin C 10% |
|---|---|---|
| Calcium 0% | • | Iron 2% |
| Thiamin 4% | • | Vitamin B6 8% |

* Percent Daily Values are based on a 2,000 calorie diet. Your daily values may be higher or lower depending on your calorie needs:

| | | Calories: | 2,000 | 2,500 |
|---|---|---|---|---|
| Total Fat | Less than | | 65g | 80g |
| Sat Fat | Less than | | 20g | 25g |
| Cholesterol | Less than | | 300mg | 300mg |
| Sodium | Less than | | 2,400mg | 2,400mg |
| Potassium | | | 3,500mg | 3,500mg |
| Total Carbohydrate | | | 300g | 375g |
| Dietary Fiber | | | 25g | 30g |

Calories per gram:
Fat 9   •   Carbohydrate 4   •   Protein 4

**Ingredients:** Potatoes, Vegetable Oil (Sunflower, Corn, and/or Canola Oil), BBQ Seasoning (Sugar, Dextrose, Salt, Malted Barley Flour, Torula Yeast, Molasses, Maltodextrin [Made From Corn], Natural Flavors [Including Natural Smoke Flavor], Spices, Paprika, Corn Starch, Tomato Powder, Garlic Powder, Yeast Extract, Onion Powder, and Paprika Extract).

Rating: 3/10 Stars

## Lays classics

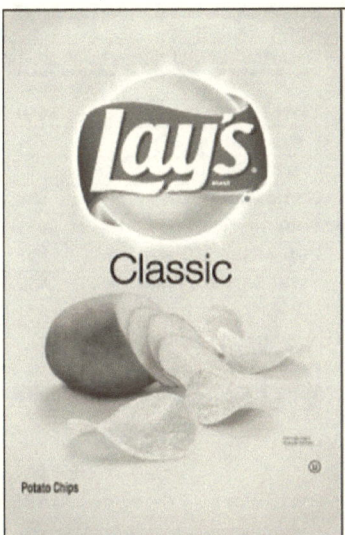

**Nutrition Facts**
Serving Size 1 oz (28g/About 15 chips)

| Amount Per Serving | |
|---|---|
| **Calories** 160 | Calories from Fat 90 |

| | % Daily Value* |
|---|---|
| **Total Fat** 10g | **16%** |
| Saturated Fat 1.5g | **8%** |
| Trans Fat 0g | |
| **Cholesterol** 0mg | **0%** |
| **Sodium** 170mg | **7%** |
| **Potassium** 350mg | **10%** |
| **Total Carbohydrate** 15g | **5%** |
| Dietary Fiber 1g | **5%** |
| Sugars less than 1g | |
| **Protein** 2g | |

| | | |
|---|---|---|
| Vitamin A 0% | • | Vitamin C 10% |
| Calcium 0% | • | Iron 2% |
| Vitamin E 6% | • | Thiamin 4% |
| Niacin 6% | • | Vitamin B₆ 10% |
| Magnesium 4% | • | Zinc 2% |

* Percent Daily Values are based on a 2,000 calorie diet. Your daily values may be higher or lower depending on your calorie needs:

| | Calories: | 2,000 | 2,500 |
|---|---|---|---|
| Total Fat | Less than | 65g | 80g |
| Sat Fat | Less than | 20g | 25g |
| Cholesterol | Less than | 300mg | 300mg |
| Sodium | Less than | 2,400mg | 2,400mg |
| Potassium | | 3,500mg | 3,500mg |
| Total Carbohydrate | | 300g | 375g |
| Dietary Fiber | | 25g | 30g |

Calories per gram:
Fat 9 • Carbohydrate 4 • Protein 4

**Ingredients:** Potatoes, Vegetable Oil (Sunflower, Corn and/or Canola Oil), and Salt.

Rating: 2.5/10 Stars

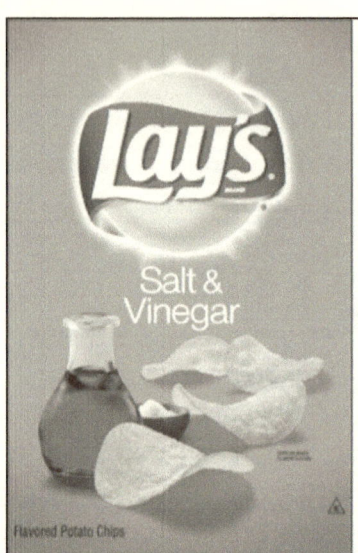

## Nutrition Facts

Serving Size 1 oz (28g/About 17 chips)

**Amount Per Serving**

**Calories** 160      Calories from Fat 90

|  | % Daily Value* |
|---|---|
| **Total Fat** 10g | **15%** |
| Saturated Fat 1.5g | **7%** |
| Trans Fat 0g | |
| **Cholesterol** 0mg | **0%** |
| **Sodium** 220mg | **9%** |
| **Potassium** 320mg | **9%** |
| **Total Carbohydrate** 15g | **5%** |
| Dietary Fiber 1g | **5%** |
| Sugars less than 1g | |
| **Protein** 2g | |

| | | |
|---|---|---|
| Vitamin A 0% | • | Vitamin C 10% |
| Calcium 0% | • | Iron 2% |
| Thiamin 4% | • | Niacin 6% |
| Phosphorus 2% | • | Magnesium 4% |

* Percent Daily Values are based on a 2,000 calorie diet. Your daily values may be higher or lower depending on your calorie needs:

| | Calories: | 2,000 | 2,500 |
|---|---|---|---|
| Total Fat | Less than | 65g | 80g |
| Sat Fat | Less than | 20g | 25g |
| Cholesterol | Less than | 300mg | 300mg |
| Sodium | Less than | 2,400mg | 2,400mg |
| Potassium | | 3,500mg | 3,500mg |
| Total Carbohydrate | | 300g | 375g |
| Dietary Fiber | | 25g | 30g |

Calories per gram:
Fat 9   •   Carbohydrate 4   •   Protein 4

**Ingredients:** Potatoes, Vegetable Oil (Sunflower, Corn and/or Canola Oil), Salt & Vinegar Seasoning (Maltodextrin [Made From Corn], Natural Flavors, Salt, Malic Acid, and Vinegar).

Rating 2/10 Star

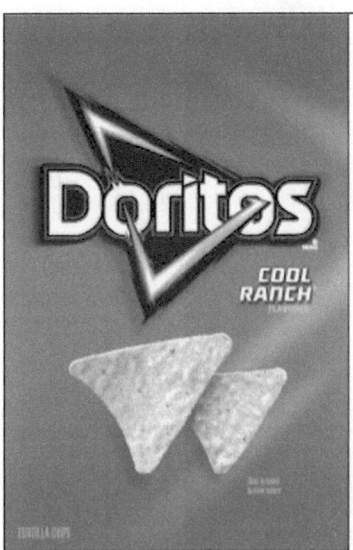

## Nutrition Facts

Serving Size 1 oz (28g/About 12 chips)

**Amount Per Serving**

**Calories** 150     Calories from Fat 70

|  | % Daily Value* |
|---|---|
| **Total Fat** 8g | **12%** |
| Saturated Fat 1g | **5%** |
| Trans Fat 0g | |
| **Cholesterol** 0mg | **0%** |
| **Sodium** 180mg | **8%** |
| **Total Carbohydrate** 18g | **6%** |
| Dietary Fiber 2g | **6%** |
| Sugars less than 1g | |
| **Protein** 2g | |

| | | |
|---|---|---|
| Vitamin A 0% | • | Vitamin C 0% |
| Calcium 2% | • | Iron 0% |
| Vitamin E 6% | • | Thiamin 4% |
| Riboflavin 2% | • | Vitamin B$_6$ 4% |
| Phosphorus 4% | • | Magnesium 4% |

\* Percent Daily Values are based on a 2,000 calorie diet. Your daily values may be higher or lower depending on your calorie needs:

| | | Calories: | 2,000 | 2,500 |
|---|---|---|---|---|
| Total Fat | Less than | | 65g | 80g |
| Sat Fat | Less than | | 20g | 25g |
| Cholesterol | Less than | | 300mg | 300mg |
| Sodium | Less than | | 2,400mg | 2,400mg |
| Total Carbohydrate | | | 300g | 375g |
| Dietary Fiber | | | 25g | 30g |

Calories per gram:
Fat 9 • Carbohydrate 4 • Protein 4

**Ingredients:** Corn, Vegetable Oil (Corn, Canola, and/or Sunflower Oil), Maltodextrin (Made From Corn), Salt, Tomato Powder, Corn Starch, Lactose, Whey, Skim Milk, Corn Syrup Solids, Onion Powder, Sugar, Garlic Powder, Monosodium Glutamate, Cheddar Cheese (Milk, Cheese Cultures, Salt, Enzymes), Dextrose, Malic Acid, Buttermilk, Natural and Artificial Flavors, Sodium Acetate, Artificial Color (Including Red 40, Blue 1, Yellow 5), Sodium Caseinate, Spice, Citric Acid, Disodium Inosinate, and Disodium Guanylate.
**CONTAINS MILK INGREDIENTS.**

More ingredeints, lower fat surprisingly, about the same carbs
Rating: 2.5/10 Stars

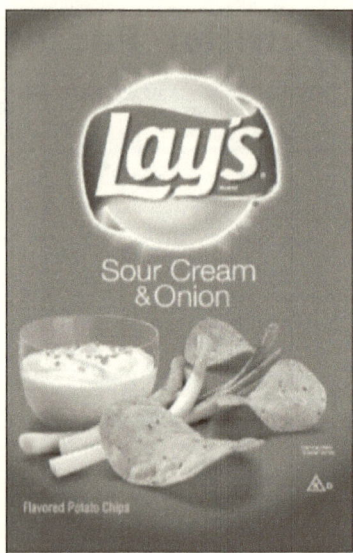

**Ingredients:** Potatoes, Vegetable Oil (Sunflower, Corn, and/or Canola Oil), Sour Cream & Onion Seasoning (Skim Milk, Salt, Maltodextrin [Made From Corn], Onion Powder, Whey, Sour Cream [Cultured Cream, Skim Milk], Canola Oil, Parsley, Natural Flavor, Lactose, Sunflower Oil, Citric Acid, Whey Protein Concentrate, and Buttermilk).
**CONTAINS MILK INGREDIENTS.**

# Nutrition Facts
Serving Size 1 oz (28g/About 17 chips)

**Amount Per Serving**

**Calories** 160      Calories from Fat 90

|  | % Daily Value* |
|---|---|
| **Total Fat** 10g | **15%** |
| Saturated Fat 1.5g | **7%** |
| Trans Fat 0g | |
| **Cholesterol** 0mg | **0%** |
| **Sodium** 160mg | **7%** |
| **Potassium** 340mg | **10%** |
| **Total Carbohydrate** 15g | **5%** |
| Dietary Fiber 1g | **5%** |
| Sugars less than 1g | |
| **Protein** 2g | |

| | | |
|---|---|---|
| Vitamin A 0% | • | Vitamin C 10% |
| Calcium 0% | • | Iron 2% |
| Vitamin E 6% | • | Thiamin 4% |
| Folate 2% | • | Magnesium 4% |

* Percent Daily Values are based on a 2,000 calorie diet. Your daily values may be higher or lower depending on your calorie needs:

| | Calories: | 2,000 | 2,500 |
|---|---|---|---|
| Total Fat | Less than | 65g | 80g |
| Sat Fat | Less than | 20g | 25g |
| Cholesterol | Less than | 300mg | 300mg |
| Sodium | Less than | 2,400mg | 2,400mg |
| Potassium | | 3,500mg | 3,500mg |
| Total Carbohydrate | | 300g | 375g |
| Dietary Fiber | | 25g | 30g |

Calories per gram:
Fat 9   •   Carbohydrate 4   •   Protein 4

Rating: 1.5/10 Stars

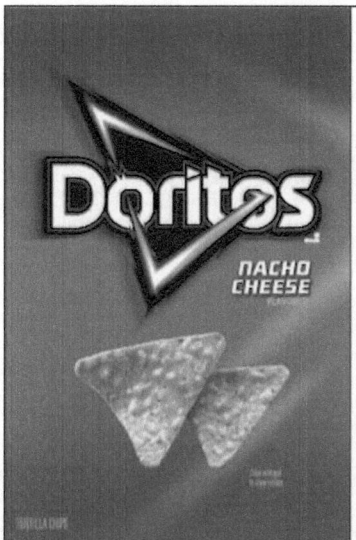

## Nutrition Facts
Serving Size 1 oz (28g/About 11 chips)

**Amount Per Serving**

**Calories** 140     Calories from Fat 70

|  | % Daily Value* |
|---|---|
| **Total Fat** 8g | **12%** |
| Saturated Fat 1g | **5%** |
| Trans Fat 0g | |
| **Cholesterol** 0mg | **0%** |
| **Sodium** 210mg | **9%** |
| **Total Carbohydrate** 16g | **5%** |
| Dietary Fiber 1g | **4%** |
| Sugars 0g | |
| **Protein** 2g | |

| | | |
|---|---|---|
| Vitamin A 2% | • | Vitamin C 0% |
| Calcium 0% | • | Iron 0% |
| Thiamin 2% | • | Vitamin B6 2% |

* Percent Daily Values are based on a 2,000 calorie diet. Your daily values may be higher or lower depending on your calorie needs:

| | | Calories: | 2,000 | 2,500 |
|---|---|---|---|---|
| Total Fat | Less than | | 65g | 80g |
| Sat Fat | Less than | | 20g | 25g |
| Cholesterol | Less than | | 300mg | 300mg |
| Sodium | Less than | | 2,400mg | 2,400mg |
| Total Carbohydrate | | | 300g | 375g |
| Dietary Fiber | | | 25g | 30g |

Calories per gram:
Fat 9 • Carbohydrate 4 • Protein 4

**Ingredients:** Corn, Vegetable Oil (Sunflower, Canola, and/or Corn Oil), Maltodextrin (Made From Corn), Salt, Cheddar Cheese (Milk, Cheese Cultures, Salt, Enzymes), Whey, Monosodium Glutamate, Buttermilk, Romano Cheese (Part-Skim Cow's Milk, Cheese Cultures, Salt, Enzymes), Whey Protein Concentrate, Onion Powder, Corn Flour, Natural and Artificial Flavor, Dextrose, Tomato Powder, Lactose, Spices, Artificial Color (Including Yellow 6, Yellow 5, and Red 40), Lactic Acid, Citric Acid, Sugar, Garlic Powder, Skim Milk, Red and Green Bell Pepper Powder, Disodium Inosinate, and Disodium Guanylate.
**CONTAINS MILK INGREDIENTS.**

**Rating: 1/10 Stars**

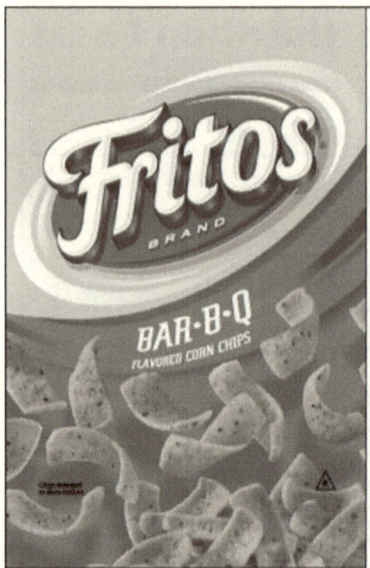

## Nutrition Facts

Serving Size 1 oz (28g/About 29 chips)

**Amount Per Serving**

**Calories** 150      Calories from Fat 90

% Daily Value*

| | |
|---|---|
| **Total Fat** 10g | **15%** |
| Saturated Fat 1.5g | **7%** |
| Trans Fat 0g | |
| Polyunsaturated Fat 6g | |
| Monounsaturated Fat 2.5g | |
| **Cholesterol** 0mg | **0%** |
| **Sodium** 290mg | **12%** |
| **Total Carbohydrate** 16g | **5%** |
| Dietary Fiber 1g | **5%** |
| Sugars less than 1g | |
| **Protein** 2g | |

| | | |
|---|---|---|
| Vitamin A 2% | • | Vitamin C 0% |
| Calcium 4% | • | Iron 2% |
| Vitamin E 6% | • | Vitamin B₆ 2% |
| Phosphorus 4% | | |

* Percent Daily Values are based on a 2,000 calorie diet. Your daily values may be higher or lower depending on your calorie needs:

| | Calories: | 2,000 | 2,500 |
|---|---|---|---|
| Total Fat | Less than | 65g | 80g |
| Sat Fat | Less than | 20g | 25g |
| Cholesterol | Less than | 300mg | 300mg |
| Sodium | Less than | 2,400mg | 2,400mg |
| Total Carbohydrate | | 300g | 375g |
| Dietary Fiber | | 25g | 30g |

Calories per gram:
Fat 9   •   Carbohydrate 4   •   Protein 4

**INGREDIENTS:** Corn, Corn Oil, Bar-B-Q Seasoning (Salt, Yellow Corn Flour, Spices, Dextrose, Sugar, Onion Powder, Monosodium Glutamate, Tomato Powder, Paprika, Modified Corn Starch, Hydrolyzed [Corn Gluten, Soy, and Wheat Gluten] Protein, Citric Acid, Extractives of Paprika, Garlic Powder, Artificial Color, Natural and Artificial Flavor, Disodium Inosinate, and Disodium Guanylate.
**CONTAINS SOY AND WHEAT INGREDIENTS.**

**Rating: 1.5/10 Stars**

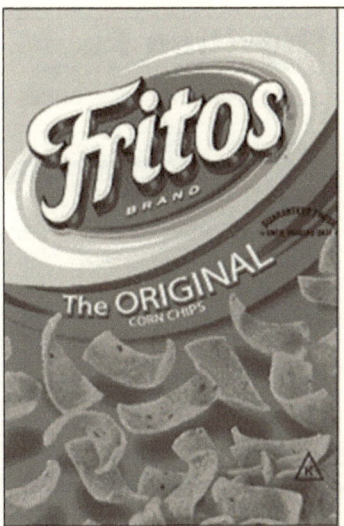

**Nutrition Facts**

Serving Size 1 oz. (28g/About 32 chips)
Servings Per Container 3

| Amount Per Serving | |
|---|---|
| **Calories** 160 | Calories from Fat 90 |

| | % Daily Value* |
|---|---|
| **Total Fat** 10g | **16%** |
| Saturated Fat 1.5g | **7%** |
| Trans Fat 0g | |
| **Cholesterol** 0mg | **0%** |
| **Sodium** 170mg | **7%** |
| **Total Carbohydrate** 15g | **5%** |
| Dietary Fiber 1g | **4%** |
| Sugars less than 1g | |
| **Protein** 2g | |

| | | | |
|---|---|---|---|
| Vitamin A 0% | • | Vitamin C 0% | |
| Calcium 2% | • | Iron 0% | |
| Vitamin E 6% | • | Vitamin B6 2% | |
| Phosphorus 4% | | | |

* Percent Daily Values are based on a 2,000 calorie diet. Your daily values may be higher or lower depending on your calorie needs:

| | | Calories: | 2,000 | 2,500 |
|---|---|---|---|---|
| Total Fat | Less than | | 65g | 80g |
| Sat Fat | Less than | | 20g | 25g |
| Cholesterol | Less than | | 300mg | 300mg |
| Sodium | Less than | | 2,400mg | 2,400mg |
| Total Carbohydrate | | | 300g | 375g |
| Dietary Fiber | | | 25g | 30g |

Calories per gram:
Fat 9 • Carbohydrate 4 • Protein 4

**INGREDIENTS:** CORN, CORN OIL, AND SALT.
NO PRESERVATIVES.

**Rating: 2/10 Stars**

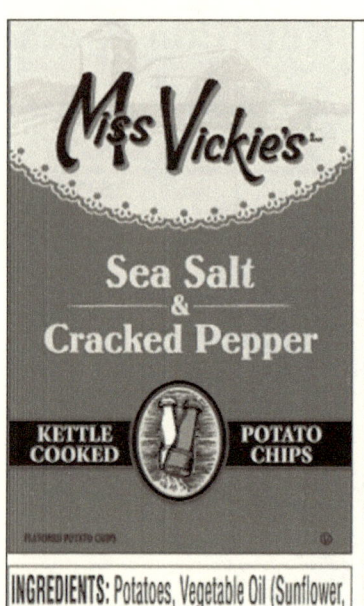

## Nutrition Facts
Serving Size 1 oz (28g/About 18 chips)

**Amount Per Serving**

**Calories** 150     Calories from Fat 80

| | % Daily Value* |
|---|---|
| **Total Fat** 9g | **14%** |
| Saturated Fat 1.5g | **9%** |
| Trans Fat 0g | |
| **Cholesterol** 0mg | **0%** |
| **Sodium** 110mg | **5%** |
| **Potassium** 360mg | **10%** |
| **Total Carbohydrate** 16g | **5%** |
| Dietary Fiber 1g | **6%** |
| Sugars less than 1g | |
| **Protein** 2g | |

| | | |
|---|---|---|
| Vitamin A 0% | • | Vitamin C 10% |
| Calcium 0% | • | Iron 4% |
| Niacin 6% | • | Vitamin B6 10% |
| Phosphorus 4% | • | Magnesium 4% |

\* Percent Daily Values are based on a 2,000 calorie diet. Your daily values may be higher or lower depending on your calorie needs:

| | Calories: | 2,000 | 2,500 |
|---|---|---|---|
| Total Fat | Less than | 65g | 80g |
| Sat Fat | Less than | 20g | 25g |
| Cholesterol | Less than | 300mg | 300mg |
| Sodium | Less than | 2,400mg | 2,400mg |
| Potassium | | 3,500mg | 3,500mg |
| Total Carbohydrate | | 300g | 375g |
| Dietary Fiber | | 25g | 30g |

Calories per gram:
Fat 9 • Carbohydrate 4 • Protein 4

**INGREDIENTS:** Potatoes, Vegetable Oil (Sunflower, Canola, and/or Corn Oil), Sea Salt & Cracked Pepper Seasoning (Maltodextrin [Made From Corn], Black Pepper, Sea Salt, Garlic Powder, Onion Powder, Natural Flavor, Sodium Citrate, and Yeast Extract).

**Rating: 3.5/10**

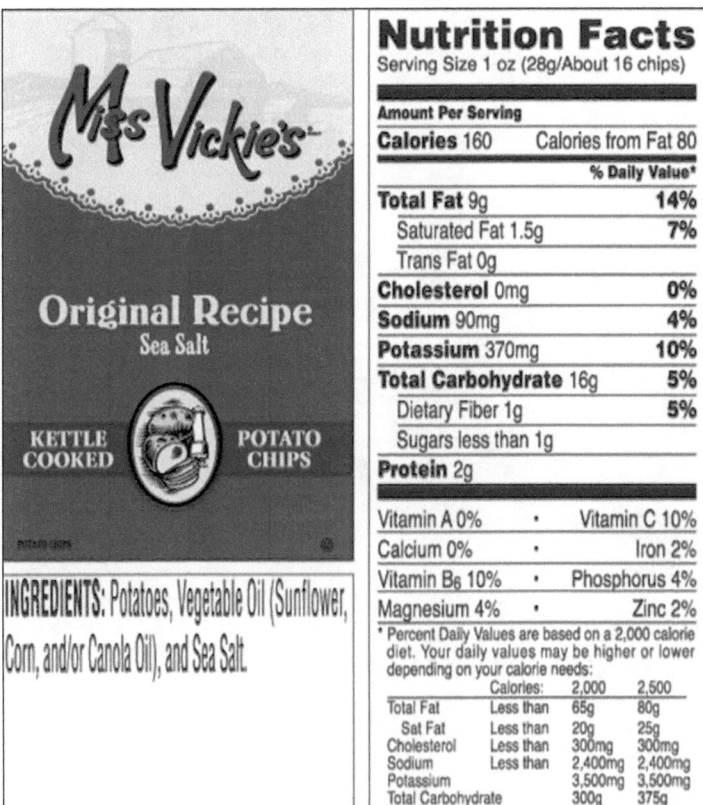

**Nutrition Facts**
Serving Size 1 oz (28g/About 16 chips)

**Amount Per Serving**

**Calories** 160      Calories from Fat 80

% Daily Value*

| | |
|---|---|
| **Total Fat** 9g | **14%** |
| Saturated Fat 1.5g | **7%** |
| Trans Fat 0g | |
| **Cholesterol** 0mg | **0%** |
| **Sodium** 90mg | **4%** |
| **Potassium** 370mg | **10%** |
| **Total Carbohydrate** 16g | **5%** |
| Dietary Fiber 1g | **5%** |
| Sugars less than 1g | |
| **Protein** 2g | |

| | | |
|---|---|---|
| Vitamin A 0% | • | Vitamin C 10% |
| Calcium 0% | • | Iron 2% |
| Vitamin B$_6$ 10% | • | Phosphorus 4% |
| Magnesium 4% | • | Zinc 2% |

* Percent Daily Values are based on a 2,000 calorie diet. Your daily values may be higher or lower depending on your calorie needs:

| | Calories: | 2,000 | 2,500 |
|---|---|---|---|
| Total Fat | Less than | 65g | 80g |
| Sat Fat | Less than | 20g | 25g |
| Cholesterol | Less than | 300mg | 300mg |
| Sodium | Less than | 2,400mg | 2,400mg |
| Potassium | | 3,500mg | 3,500mg |
| Total Carbohydrate | | 300g | 375g |
| Dietary Fiber | | 25g | 30g |

Calories per gram:
Fat 9 • Carbohydrate 4 • Protein 4

**Original Recipe**
Sea Salt

KETTLE COOKED     POTATO CHIPS

**INGREDIENTS:** Potatoes, Vegetable Oil (Sunflower, Corn, and/or Canola Oil), and Sea Salt.

**Rating: 3.5/10**

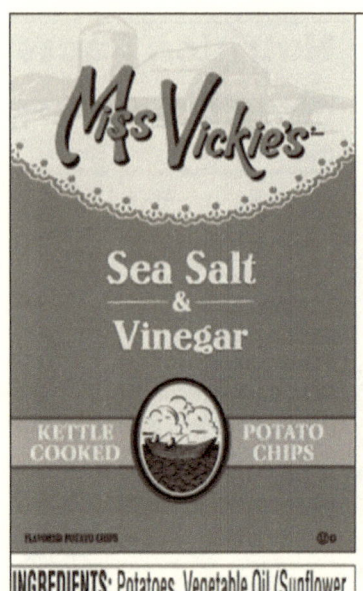

**INGREDIENTS:** Potatoes, Vegetable Oil (Sunflower, Canola, and/or Corn Oil,) Sea Salt & Vinegar Seasoning (Maltodextrin [Made From Corn], Sea Salt, Vinegar, Buttermilk, Lactose, Sugar, Dextrose, Yeast Extract, Citric Acid, and Sunflower Oil).
**CONTAINS MILK INGREDIENTS.**

# Nutrition Facts

Serving Size 1 oz (28g/About 18 chips)

**Amount Per Serving**

**Calories** 150      Calories from Fat 80

| | % Daily Value* |
|---|---|
| **Total Fat** 9g | **13%** |
| Saturated Fat 1.5g | **6%** |
| Trans Fat 0g | |
| **Cholesterol** 0mg | **0%** |
| **Sodium** 170mg | **7%** |
| **Potassium** 340mg | **10%** |
| **Total Carbohydrate** 17g | **6%** |
| Dietary Fiber 1g | **5%** |
| Sugars 1g | |
| **Protein** 2g | |

| | | |
|---|---|---|
| Vitamin A 0% | • | Vitamin C 10% |
| Calcium 0% | • | Iron 2% |
| Thiamin 4% | • | Vitamin B6 10% |
| Magnesium 4% | • | Zinc 2% |

* Percent Daily Values are based on a 2,000 calorie diet. Your daily values may be higher or lower depending on your calorie needs:

| | Calories: | 2,000 | 2,500 |
|---|---|---|---|
| Total Fat | Less than | 65g | 80g |
| Sat Fat | Less than | 20g | 25g |
| Cholesterol | Less than | 300mg | 300mg |
| Sodium | Less than | 2,400mg | 2,400mg |
| Potassium | | 3,500mg | 3,500mg |
| Total Carbohydrate | | 300g | 375g |
| Dietary Fiber | | 25g | 30g |

Calories per gram:
Fat 9  •  Carbohydrate 4  •  Protein 4

Rating: 2/10

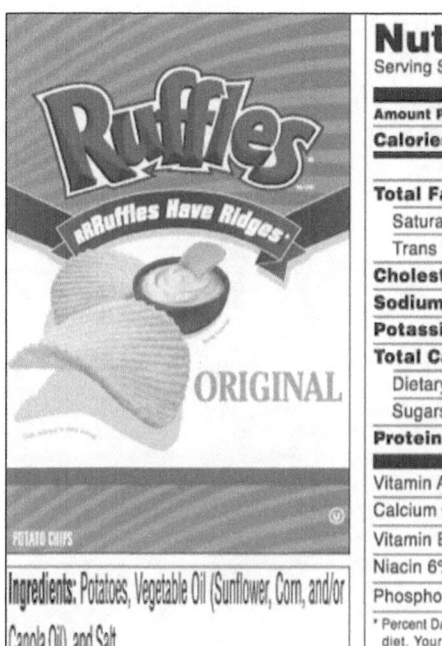

## Nutrition Facts

Serving Size 1 oz (28g/About 12 chips)

**Amount Per Serving**

| **Calories** 160 | Calories from Fat 90 |
|---|---|

| | % Daily Value* |
|---|---|
| **Total Fat** 10g | **16%** |
| Saturated Fat 1.5g | **7%** |
| Trans Fat 0g | |
| **Cholesterol** 0mg | **0%** |
| **Sodium** 160mg | **7%** |
| **Potassium** 340mg | **10%** |
| **Total Carbohydrate** 15g | **5%** |
| Dietary Fiber 1g | **5%** |
| Sugars less than 1g | |
| **Protein** 2g | |

| | | |
|---|---|---|
| Vitamin A 0% | • | Vitamin C 10% |
| Calcium 0% | • | Iron 2% |
| Vitamin E 6% | • | Thiamin 4% |
| Niacin 6% | • | Vitamin B₆ 10% |
| Phosphorus 2% | • | Magnesium 4% |

* Percent Daily Values are based on a 2,000 calorie diet. Your daily values may be higher or lower depending on your calorie needs:

| | Calories: | 2,000 | 2,500 |
|---|---|---|---|
| Total Fat | Less than | 65g | 80g |
| Sat Fat | Less than | 20g | 25g |
| Cholesterol | Less than | 300mg | 300mg |
| Sodium | Less than | 2,400mg | 2,400mg |
| Potassium | | 3,500mg | 3,500mg |
| Total Carbohydrate | | 300g | 375g |
| Dietary Fiber | | 25g | 30g |

Calories per gram:
Fat 9 • Carbohydrate 4 • Protein 4

Rating: 2.5/10

# Pringles Original

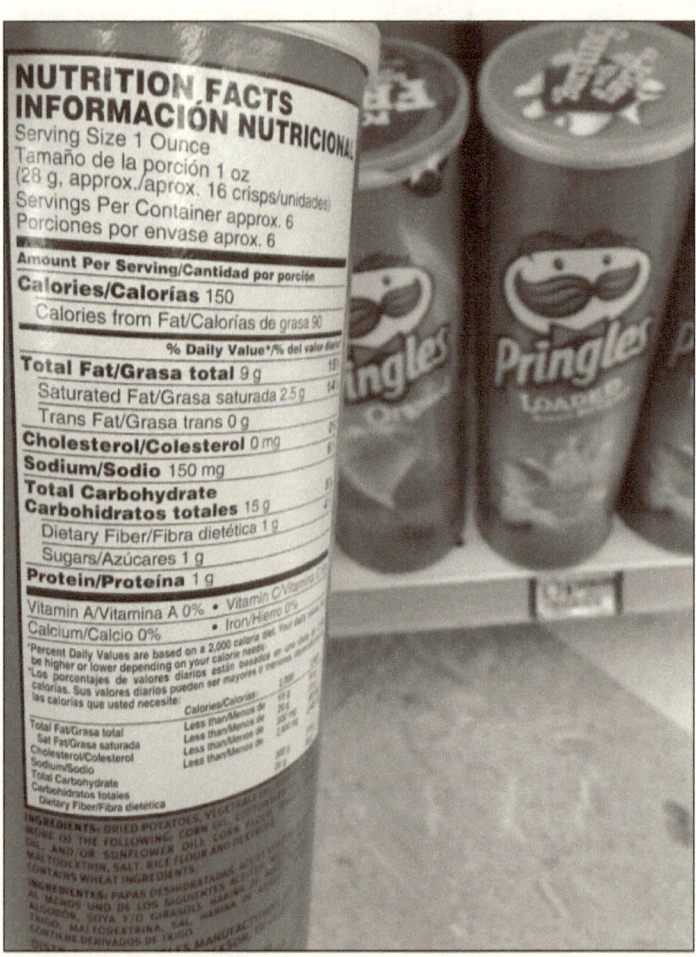

**Rating:1.5/10**

# Kettle Brand® Potato Chips
## Sea Salt

**Ingredients:** Potatoes, safflower and/or sunflower and/or canola oil, sea salt.

**United States:**

**Canada:**

## Nutrition Facts

Serving Size 1oz about 13 chips (28g)
Servings Per Container

Amount Per Serving

| Calories 150 | Calories from Fat 80 |
|---|---|
| | **% Daily Value\*** |
| **Total Fat** 9g | **14%** |
| Saturated Fat 1g | **5%** |
| Trans Fat 0g | |
| Polyunsaturated Fat 1g | |
| Monounsaturated Fat 7g | |
| **Cholesterol** 0mg | **0%** |
| **Sodium** 115mg | **5%** |
| **Potassium** 430mg | **12%** |
| **Total Carbohydrate** 16g | **5%** |
| Dietary Fiber 1g | **4%** |
| Sugars 0g | |
| **Protein** 2g | |

| Vitamin A 0% | • | Vitamin C 10% |
|---|---|---|
| Calcium 0% | • | Iron 2% |

\*Percent Daily Values are based on a 2,000 calorie diet. Your daily values may be higher or lower depending on your calorie needs:

| | | Calories: | 2,000 | 2,500 |
|---|---|---|---|---|
| Total Fat | Less than | | 65g | 80g |
| Saturated Fat | Less than | | 20g | 25g |
| Cholesterol | Less than | | 300mg | 300mg |
| Sodium | Less than | | 2,400mg | 2,400mg |
| Potassium | | | 3,500 mg | 3,500 mg |
| Total Carbohydrate | | | 300g | 375g |
| Dietary Fiber | | | 25g | 30g |

Calories per gram:
Fat 9 • Carbohydrate 4 • Protein 4

## Nutrition Facts
## Valeur nutritive

Serving Size 18-20 chips (40 g)
Portion (40 g)

| Amount<br>Teneur | % Daily Value<br>% valeur quotidienne |
|---|---|
| **Calories / Calories** 210 | |
| **Fat / Lipides** 13 g | **20 %** |
| Saturated Fat / Lipides saturés 1 g<br>+ Trans Fat / lipides trans 0 g | **5 %** |
| **Cholesterol / Cholestérol** 0 mg | |
| **Sodium / Sodium** 160 mg | **7 %** |
| **Carbohydrate / Glucides** 22 g | **7 %** |
| Fibre / Fibres 2 g | **8 %** |
| Sugars / Sucres 0 g | |
| **Protein / Protéines** 3 g | |
| Vitamin A / Vitamine A | 0 % |
| Vitamin C / Vitamine C | 15 % |
| Calcium / Calcium | 0 % |
| Iron / Fer | 4 % |

Rating: 4.5/10

# Kettle Brand® Potato Chips
## Unsalted (United States only)
## Low Sodium (Canada only)

**Ingredients:** Potatoes, safflower and/or sunflower and/or canola oil.

**United States:**

## Nutrition Facts

Serving Size 1oz about 13 chips (28g)
Servings Per Container

Amount Per Serving

| | |
|---|---|
| **Calories** 150 | Calories from Fat 80 |

| | % Daily Value* |
|---|---|
| **Total Fat** 9g | **14%** |
| Saturated Fat 1g | **5%** |
| Trans Fat 0g | |
| Polyunsaturated Fat 1g | |
| Monounsaturated Fat 7g | |
| **Cholesterol** 0mg | **0%** |
| **Sodium** 5mg | **0%** |
| **Potassium** 440mg | **13%** |
| **Total Carbohydrate** 16g | **5%** |
| Dietary Fiber 2g | **8%** |
| Sugars 0g | |
| **Protein** 2g | |

| | | |
|---|---|---|
| Vitamin A 0% | • | Vitamin C 10% |
| Calcium 0% | • | Iron 2% |

*Percent Daily Values are based on a 2,000 calorie diet. Your daily values may be higher or lower depending on your calorie needs:

| | | Calories: | 2,000 | 2,500 |
|---|---|---|---|---|
| Total Fat | Less than | | 65g | 80g |
| Saturated Fat | Less than | | 20g | 25g |
| Cholesterol | Less than | | 300mg | 300mg |
| Sodium | Less than | | 2,400mg | 2,400mg |
| Potassium | | | 3,500 mg | 3,500 mg |
| Total Carbohydrate | | | 300g | 375g |
| Dietary Fiber | | | 25g | 30g |

Calories per gram:
Fat 9 • Carbohydrate 4 • Protein 4

**Canada:**

## Nutrition Facts
## Valeur nutritive

Serving Size 18-20 chips (40 g)
Portion (40 g)

| Amount<br>Teneur | % Daily Value<br>% valeur quotidienne |
|---|---|
| **Calories / Calories** 220 | |
| **Fat / Lipides** 13 g | **20 %** |
| Saturated Fat / Lipides saturés 1 g<br>+ Trans Fat / lipides trans 0 g | **5 %** |
| **Cholesterol / Cholestérol** 0 mg | |
| **Sodium / Sodium** 10 mg | **1 %** |
| **Carbohydrate / Glucides** 23 g | **8 %** |
| Fibre / Fibres 2 g | **8 %** |
| Sugars / Sucres 0 g | |
| **Protein / Protéines** 3 g | |
| Vitamin A / Vitamine A | **0 %** |
| Vitamin C / Vitamine C | **15 %** |
| Calcium / Calcium | **0 %** |
| Iron / Fer | **4 %** |

Rating:4/10

# Pop chips Originals

share bag (3.5 oz.)

**nutrition facts.**

**serving size 1oz** (28g/about 23 chips)
servings per container 3.5

| | |
|---|---|
| **calories** 120  calories from fat 35 | |
| | % daily value |
| **total fat** 4g | 6% |
| saturated fat 0g | 0% |
| trans fat 0g | |
| polyunsaturated fat 0.5g | |
| monounsaturated fat 3g | |
| **cholesterol** 0mg | 0% |
| **sodium** 190mg | 8% |
| **potassium** 140mg | 4% |
| **total carbohydrate** 19g | 6% |
| dietary fiber 1g | 4% |
| sugars 0g | |
| **protein** 1g | |

**ingredients:**
dried potato, rice flour, sunflower, safflower, and/or canola oil, potato starch, sea salt, salt.

Rating:4/10 stars

# Pop chips Sea Salt

share bag (4 oz.)
**nutrition facts.**

**serving size 1oz** (28g/about 15 chips)
servings per container 4

| | |
|---|---|
| **calories** 130 | calories from fat 50 |

| | % daily value |
|---|---|
| **total fat** 5g | 8% |
| saturated fat 0.5g | 3% |
| trans fat 0g | |
| polyunsaturated fat 1g | |
| monounsaturated fat 3g | |
| **cholesterol** 0mg | 0% |
| **sodium** 200mg | 8% |
| **total carbohydrate** 18g | 6% |
| dietary fiber 2g | 8% |
| sugars 1g | |
| **protein** 2g | |

**ingredients:**
stone-ground whole corn masa treated with lime, sunflower, safflower, and/or canola oil, seasoning (salt, buttermilk powder, whey powder, tomato powder, onion powder, sugar, garlic powder, cheddar cheese [milk, cultures, salt, enzymes], autolyzed yeast extract, dehydrated butter [cream, salt], corn malto-dextrin, spice, nonfat dry milk, natural flavors, annatto, citric acid, paprika oleoresin [color], dried milkfat, turmeric),

Rating: 4.5/10 stars

## Tostitoes simply natural

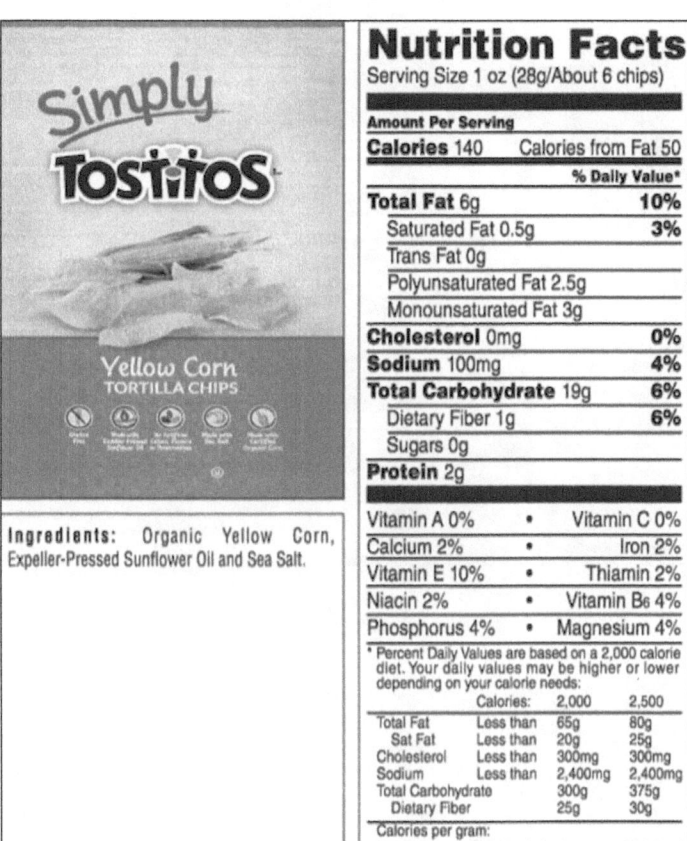

**Nutrition Facts**
Serving Size 1 oz (28g/About 6 chips)

| Amount Per Serving | |
| --- | --- |
| **Calories** 140 | Calories from Fat 50 |

| | % Daily Value* |
| --- | --- |
| **Total Fat** 6g | **10%** |
| Saturated Fat 0.5g | **3%** |
| Trans Fat 0g | |
| Polyunsaturated Fat 2.5g | |
| Monounsaturated Fat 3g | |
| **Cholesterol** 0mg | **0%** |
| **Sodium** 100mg | **4%** |
| **Total Carbohydrate** 19g | **6%** |
| Dietary Fiber 1g | **6%** |
| Sugars 0g | |
| **Protein** 2g | |

| | | |
| --- | --- | --- |
| Vitamin A 0% | • | Vitamin C 0% |
| Calcium 2% | • | Iron 2% |
| Vitamin E 10% | • | Thiamin 2% |
| Niacin 2% | • | Vitamin B6 4% |
| Phosphorus 4% | • | Magnesium 4% |

* Percent Daily Values are based on a 2,000 calorie diet. Your daily values may be higher or lower depending on your calorie needs:

| | | Calories: | 2,000 | 2,500 |
| --- | --- | --- | --- | --- |
| Total Fat | Less than | | 65g | 80g |
| Sat Fat | Less than | | 20g | 25g |
| Cholesterol | Less than | | 300mg | 300mg |
| Sodium | Less than | | 2,400mg | 2,400mg |
| Total Carbohydrate | | | 300g | 375g |
| Dietary Fiber | | | 25g | 30g |

Calories per gram:
Fat 9 • Carbohydrate 4 • Protein 4

**Ingredients:** Organic Yellow Corn, Expeller-Pressed Sunflower Oil and Sea Salt.

Rating: 3/10 stars

# Tostitos Restaurant Original

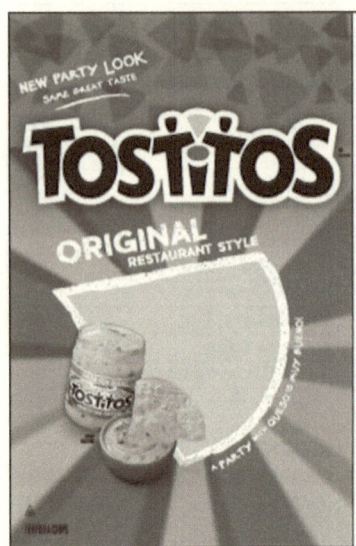

**INGREDIENTS:** Corn, Vegetable Oil (Corn, Canola and/or Sunflower Oil), and Salt.

No Preservatives.

## Nutrition Facts
Serving Size 1 oz (28g/About 7 chips)

**Amount Per Serving**

| | |
|---|---|
| **Calories** 140 | Calories from Fat 60 |

**% Daily Value\***

| | |
|---|---|
| **Total Fat** 7g | **10%** |
| Saturated Fat 1g | **5%** |
| Trans Fat 0g | |
| **Cholesterol** 0mg | **0%** |
| **Sodium** 115mg | **5%** |
| **Total Carbohydrate** 19g | **6%** |
| Dietary Fiber 1g | **5%** |
| Sugars 0g | |
| **Protein** 2g | |

| | | |
|---|---|---|
| Vitamin A 0% | • | Vitamin C 0% |
| Calcium 2% | • | Iron 2% |

\* Percent Daily Values are based on a 2,000 calorie diet. Your daily values may be higher or lower depending on your calorie needs:

| | | Calories: | 2,000 | 2,500 |
|---|---|---|---|---|
| Total Fat | Less than | | 65g | 80g |
| Sat Fat | Less than | | 20g | 25g |
| Cholesterol | Less than | | 300mg | 300mg |
| Sodium | Less than | | 2,400mg | 2,400mg |
| Total Carbohydrate | | | 300g | 375g |
| Dietary Fiber | | | 25g | 30g |

Calories per gram:
Fat 9 • Carbohydrate 4 • Protein 4

Rating: 3/10 Stars

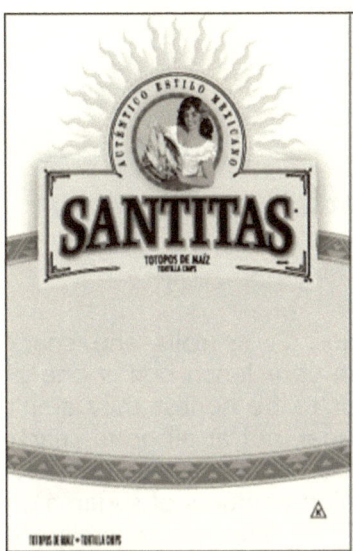

**Información Nutrimental
Nutrition Facts**

Tamaño de una Porción 1 onza (28g/aprox. 9 totopos)
Serving Size 1 oz (28g/About 9 chips)

| Cantidad por Porción / Amount Per Serving | |
|---|---|
| **Calorías** 140 | Calorías de Grasa 50 |
| **Calories** 140 | Calories from Fat 50 |
| | % Valor Diario* / % Daily Value* |
| **Grasas Totales / Total Fat** 6g | **9%** |
| Grasa Saturada / Saturated Fat 1g | **5%** |
| Grasa Trans / Trans Fat 0g | |
| **Colesterol / Cholesterol** 0mg | **0%** |
| **Sodio / Sodium** 115mg | **5%** |
| **Carbohidratos Totales** 19g | **6%** |
| **Total Carbohydrate** 19g | **6%** |
| Fibra Dietética / Dietary Fiber 2g | **7%** |
| Azúcares / Sugars 0g | |
| **Proteína / Protein** 2g | |

| | | |
|---|---|---|
| Vitamina A/Vitamin A 0% | • | Vitamina C/Vitamin C 0% |
| Calcio/Calcium 2% | • | Hierro/Iron 2% |

\* Los porcentajes de los valores diarios están basados en una dieta de 2,000 calorías. Sus valores diarios pueden ser mayores o menores dependiendo de su necesidad calórica:
\* Percent Daily Values are based on a 2,000 calorie diet. Your daily values may be higher or lower depending on your calorie needs:

| | | Calorías/Calories: | 2,000 | 2,500 |
|---|---|---|---|---|
| Grasas Totales/Total Fat | Menos de/Less than | | 65g | 80g |
| Grasa Saturadas/Sat Fat | Menos de/Less than | | 20g | 25g |
| Colesterol/Cholesterol | Menos de/Less than | | 300mg | 300mg |
| Sodio/Sodium | Menos de/Less than | | 2,400mg | 2,400mg |
| Carbohidratos Totales/Total Carbohydrate | | | 300g | 375g |
| Fibra Dietética/Dietary Fiber | | | 25g | 30g |

Calorías por Gramo/Calories per Gram:
Grasas/Fat 9 • Carbohidratos/Carbohydrate 4 • Proteína/Protein 4

**Ingredientes**: Maíz, Aceite Vegetal (Aceite de Maíz, Girasol, y/o Canola), y Sal.
No Contiene Conservadores.

**Ingredients**: Corn, Vegetable Oil (Corn, Sunflower, and/or Canola), and Salt.
No Preservatives.

**GLUTEN FREE**

Rating: 6/10 Stars

## Winner

Sanitas Chips

While one cannot be overly simplistic, in general, chips are not a good snack. They contain potato which is starch, salt, and mostly are fried in unhealthy oil. Their only redeeming quality is that there are usually not too many other chemicals and they are a reasonable source of potassium.

# Cakes

Everybody loves Twinkies, Swiss rolls and snack cakes. Finding a Swiss roll in your lunch box is one of the precious joys of life, but to be honest they aren't good for you. Lots of fat, sugar, not at all good snack, in general should be eaten as occasionally as possible. Snack cakes normally have high amounts of sugar, high calories, low fiber, low protein, high fat and generally are a nutritional disaster that should be enjoyed periodically

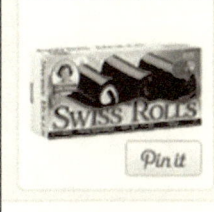

# Swiss Rolls
swiss rolls

**D-**
Grade

**270**
Calories

Pin it

# Nutrition Facts
Serving Size 2 cakes (62 g)

| Per Serving | % Daily Value* |
|---|---|
| Calories 270 | |
| Calories from Fat 108 | |
| Total Fat 12g | 18% |
| Saturated Fat 6g | 30% |
| Cholesterol 15mg | 5% |
| Sodium 140mg | 6% |
| Carbohydrates 39g | 13% |
| Dietary Fiber 0.7g | 3% |
| Sugars 26g | |
| Protein 2g | |

Vitamin A 0% · Vitamin C 0%

Calcium 0% · Iron 4%

High fat, High carbs

Rating: 3/10 Stars

# Twinkies
twinkie, snack, sweets, dessert, twinkie's

| | |
|---|---|
| **D-** | **270** |
| Grade | Calories |

## Nutrition Facts
Serving Size 2 cake (77 g)

| Per Serving | % Daily Value* |
|---|---|
| Calories 270 | |
| Calories from Fat 81 | |
| Total Fat 9g | 14% |
| Saturated Fat 4.5g | 23% |
| Cholesterol 35mg | 12% |
| Sodium 360mg | 15% |
| Carbohydrates 46g | 15% |
| Dietary Fiber 0g | 0% |
| Sugars 33g | |
| Protein 2g | |

Vitamin A 0% · Vitamin C 0%

Calcium 2% · Iron 4%

Rating: 2/10 Stars

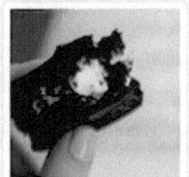

# Hostess Ding Dongs, Chocolate Cake

With Creme Filling
ding dongs, snack, dessert

**D-**
Grade

**368**
Calories

## Nutrition Facts
Serving Size 1 serving (80 g)

| Per Serving | % Daily Value* |
|---|---|
| Calories 368 | |
| Calories from Fat 174 | |
| Total Fat 19.4g | 30% |
| Saturated Fat 11g | 55% |
| Polyunsaturated Fat 1.2g | |
| Monounsaturated Fat 4g | |
| Cholesterol 14mg | 5% |
| Sodium 241mg | 10% |
| Potassium 0mg | 0% |
| Carbohydrates 45.4g | 15% |
| Dietary Fiber 1.8g | 7% |
| Sugars 32.4g | |
| Protein 3.1g | |

Vitamin A 0% · Vitamin C 0%
Calcium 0% · Iron 10%

**High calorie, high sodium, high carb, very unhealthy, surprisingly enough it does have nearly 2 grams of sugar and 3 grams of protein, very high fat**

**Rating: 4/10 Stars**

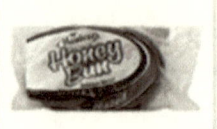

# Glazed Honey Bun
honey bun

| D | 440 |
|---|---|
| Grade | Calories |

# Nutrition Facts
Serving Size 1 bun (106 g)

| Per Serving | % Daily Value* |
|---|---:|
| **Calories** 440 | |
| Calories from Fat 225 | |
| **Total Fat** 25g | 38% |
| Saturated Fat 14g | 70% |
| **Cholesterol** 5mg | 2% |
| **Sodium** 340mg | 14% |
| **Carbohydrates** 51g | 17% |
| Dietary Fiber 1g | 4% |
| Sugars 29g | |
| **Protein** 4g | |

Vitamin A 0% · Vitamin C 0%

Calcium 15% · Iron 8%

**Rating: 3/10 stars**

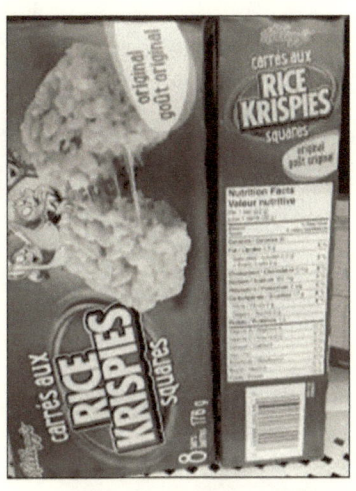

Cereal (rice, sugar, salt, corn and barley malt extract, monoglycerides, vitamins [niacinamide, folic acid], iron, colour), sugar/glucose-fructose, modified milk ingredients, corn syrup solids, fructose, palm kernel and palm oil, soybean and palm oil shortening, icing sugar, cocoa, glycerin, hydrogenated palm kernel oil, dextrose, maltodextrin, natural and artificial flavour, soy lecithin, salt, agar, sodium phosphate, polysorbate 60, bht.

## Nutrition Facts

| | |
|---|---|
| Per 1 bar / pour 1 barre | 22 g |
| Calories / Calories | 90 |
| Fat / Lipides | 2.5 g |
| Sodium / Sodium | 105 mg |
| Carbohydrate | 17 g |
| Fibre | 0 g |
| Sugars | 8 g |
| Protein | 1 g |

Rating: 2/10

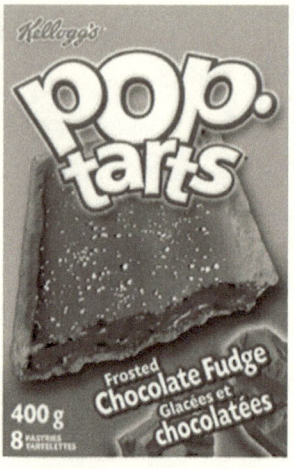

Q Enlarge

⊞ Add to Compare

| Nutrition Facts | Toas |
| --- | --- |
| Per 1 pastry / pour 1 tartelette | 50 g |
| Calories / Calories | 200 |
| Fat / Lipides | 5 g |
| Sodium / Sodium | 220 mg |
| Sugars / Sucres | 19 g |
| Fibre / Fibres | 1 g |

Q View Full Nutrition Facts panel

Wheat flour, sugar/glucose-fructose, dextrose, vegetable shortening (contains palm oil), icing sugar, modified milk ingredients, crackermeal, cocoa, modified corn starch, salt, baking powder, monoglycerides, sodium stearoyl lactylate, gelatin, dried egg whites, acetylated tartaric acid esters of mono and diglycerides, xanthan gum, natural flavour, soy lecithin, calcium phosphate, colour.

**Rating: 2.5 Stars**

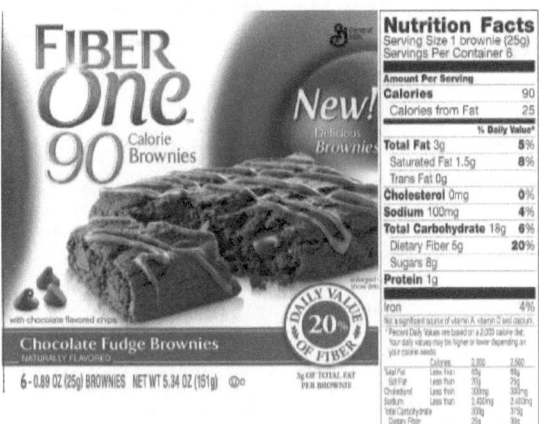

## Rating: 4/10 Stars

## Winner: Fibre 1 Brownie

### Gummies/Candies

Ever since Haribo introduced gummi bears, gummies and candy have been a staple of most childrens lunch boxes. They come in all shapes, sizes and flavours, however, if there is forum that they don't come in its healthy. Characteristically they normally have very high sugar and not much else. They are composed of a slurry of chemicals that are the farthest thing from wholesome.

# Betty Crocker Fruit Roll-Ups Strawberry & Berry Berry Cool Fruit Flavored Snacks, 0.5 oz, 20 count

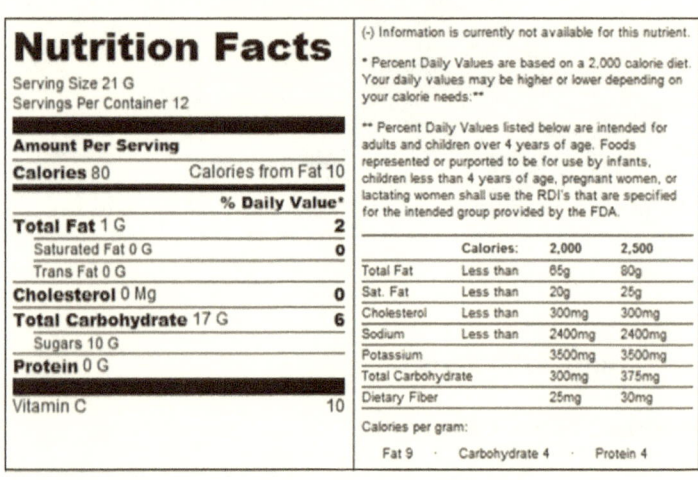

## Nutrition Facts

Serving Size 21 G
Servings Per Container 12

**Amount Per Serving**

**Calories** 80 — Calories from Fat 10

| | % Daily Value* |
|---|---|
| **Total Fat** 1 G | 2 |
| Saturated Fat 0 G | 0 |
| Trans Fat 0 G | |
| **Cholesterol** 0 Mg | 0 |
| **Total Carbohydrate** 17 G | 6 |
| Sugars 10 G | |
| **Protein** 0 G | |
| Vitamin C | 10 |

(-) Information is currently not available for this nutrient.

* Percent Daily Values are based on a 2,000 calorie diet. Your daily values may be higher or lower depending on your calorie needs:**

** Percent Daily Values listed below are intended for adults and children over 4 years of age. Foods represented or purported to be for use by infants, children less than 4 years of age, pregnant women, or lactating women shall use the RDI's that are specified for the intended group provided by the FDA.

| | | Calories: | 2,000 | 2,500 |
|---|---|---|---|---|
| Total Fat | Less than | | 65g | 80g |
| Sat. Fat | Less than | | 20g | 25g |
| Cholesterol | Less than | | 300mg | 300mg |
| Sodium | Less than | | 2400mg | 2400mg |
| Potassium | | | 3500mg | 3500mg |
| Total Carbohydrate | | | 300mg | 375mg |
| Dietary Fiber | | | 25mg | 30mg |

Calories per gram:

Fat 9  ·  Carbohydrate 4  ·  Protein 4

Strawberry Ingredients: Pears From Concentrate, Corn Syrup, Dried Corn Syrup, Sugar, Partially Hydrogenated Cottonseed Oil, Citric Acid, Sodium Citrate, Acetylated Mono And Diglycerides, Pectin, Malic Acid, Natural Flavor, Vitamin C (Ascorbic Acid), Color (Red 40, Yellows 5 % 6, Blue 1). Berry Berry Cool Ingredients: Pears From Concentrate, Corn Syrup, Dried Corn Syrup, Sugar, Partially

Hydrogenated Cottonseed Oil, Citric Acid, Sodium Citrate, Acetylated Mono And Diglycerides, Pectin, Malic Acid, Vitamin C (Ascorbic Acid), Natural And Artificial Flavor, Color (Red 40, Yellow 5, Blue 1).

**high calorie, high sugar**
**Rating:2/10**

# Betty Crocker Fruit Gushers Strawberry Splash & Tropical Flavors Variety Pack Fruit Flavored Snacks, 0.9 oz, 12 count

Tropical Flavors Ingredients: Pears From Concentrate, Sugar, Dried Corn Syrup, Corn Syrup, Modified Corn Starch, Fructose, Partially Hydrogenated Cottonseed Oil And/Or Cottonseed Oil, Grape Juice From Concentrate, Contains 2% Or Less Of: Maltodextrin, Carrageenan, Citric Acid, Glycerin, Distilled Monoglycerides, Sodium Citrate, Malic Acid, Vitamin C (Ascorbic Acid), Potassium Citrate, Agar-Agar, Natural And Artificial Flavor, Xanthan Gum, Colors (Blue 1, Yellows 5 & 6)./Strawberry Splash Ingredients: Pears From Conentrate, Sugar, Dried Corn Syrup, Corn Syrup, Modified Corn Starch, Fructose, Partially Hydrogentated, Cottonseed Oil And/Or Cottonseed Oil, Grape Juice From Concentrate. Contains 2% Or Less Of: Maltodextrin, Carrageenan, Citric Acid, Glycerin, Distilled Monoglycerides, Sodium Citrate, Malic Acid, Vitamin C (Ascorbic Acid), Natural Flavor, Potassium Citrate, Agar-Agar, Xanthan Gum, Color (Red 40, Blue 1)

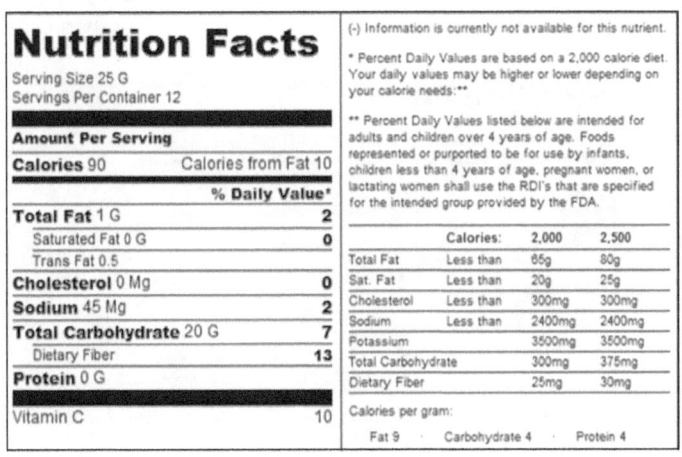

# Nutrition Facts

Serving Size 25 G
Servings Per Container 12

**Amount Per Serving**

| Calories 90 | Calories from Fat 10 |
| --- | --- |

| | % Daily Value* |
| --- | --- |
| **Total Fat** 1 G | 2 |
| Saturated Fat 0 G | 0 |
| Trans Fat 0.5 | |
| **Cholesterol** 0 Mg | 0 |
| **Sodium** 45 Mg | 2 |
| **Total Carbohydrate** 20 G | 7 |
| Dietary Fiber | 13 |
| **Protein** 0 G | |
| Vitamin C | 10 |

(-) Information is currently not available for this nutrient.

* Percent Daily Values are based on a 2,000 calorie diet. Your daily values may be higher or lower depending on your calorie needs:**

** Percent Daily Values listed below are intended for adults and children over 4 years of age. Foods represented or purported to be for use by infants, children less than 4 years of age, pregnant women, or lactating women shall use the RDI's that are specified for the intended group provided by the FDA.

| | Calories: | 2,000 | 2,500 |
| --- | --- | --- | --- |
| Total Fat | Less than | 65g | 80g |
| Sat. Fat | Less than | 20g | 25g |
| Cholesterol | Less than | 300mg | 300mg |
| Sodium | Less than | 2400mg | 2400mg |
| Potassium | | 3500mg | 3500mg |
| Total Carbohydrate | | 300mg | 375mg |
| Dietary Fiber | | 25mg | 30mg |

Calories per gram:
Fat 9  ·  Carbohydrate 4  ·  Protein 4

High carb, sodium present

Rating:3/10 Stars

# Betty Crocker Party Pack Fruit Flavored Snacks, 24 count, 9.96 oz

Fruit By The Foot: Pears from Concentrate, Sugar, Maltodextrin, Corn Syrup, Partially Hydrogenated Cottonseed Oil. Contains 2% Or Less of: Carrageenan, Citric Acid, Acetylated Monoglycerides, Sodium Citrate, Malic Acid, Xanthan Gum, Locust Bean Gum, Vitamin C (Ascorbic Acid), Potassium Citrate, Natural Flavor, Color (Yellow 5, Red 40, Blue 1). Fruit Roll-Ups: Pears from Concentrate, Corn Syrup, Dried Corn Syrup, Sugar, Partially Hydrogenated Cottonseed Oil. Contains 2% Or Less of: Citric Acid, Sodium Citrate, Acetylated Monoglycerides, Fruit Pectin, Dextrose, Malic Acid, Vitamin C (Ascorbic Acid), Natural Flavor, Color (Red 40, Yellows 5 & 6, Blue 1). Fruit Gushers: Pears from Concentrate, Sugar, Dried Corn Syrup, Corn Syrup, Modified Corn Starch, Fructose, Grape Juice from Concentrate. Contains 2% Or Less of: Partially Hydrogenated Cottonseed Oil, Maltodextrin, Cottonseed Oil, Carrageenan, Citric Acid, Glycerin, Monoglycerides, Sodium Citrate, Malic Acid, Vitamin C (Ascorbic Acid), Natural Flavor, Potassium Citrate, Agar-Agar, Color (Red 40, Blue 1, Yellows 5 & 6 And Other Color Added), Xanthan Gum.

## Nutrition Facts

Serving Size 12 G
Servings Per Container 10

| Amount Per Serving | 1 Pouch Fruit By The Foot | 1 Pouch Fruit Roll-Ups |
|---|---|---|
| **Calories** | 45 | 40 |
| Calories from Fat | 5 | 5 |
| | **% Daily Value*** | |
| **Total Fat** 0.5 G | 1 | 1 |
| Saturated Fat 0 G | 0 | 0 |
| Trans Fat 0 G | | |
| **Cholesterol** 0 Mg | 0 | 0 |
| **Sodium** 30 Mg | 1 | 2 |
| **Total Carbohydrate** 10 Mg | 3 | 3 |
| Dietary Fiber 0 G | 0 | 0 |
| Sugars 6 G | | |
| **Protein** 0 G | | |
| Vitamin A | 0 | 0 |
| Vitamin C | 6 | 6 |
| Calcium | 0 | 0 |

(-) Information is currently not available for this nutrient.

* Percent Daily Values are based on a 2,000 calorie diet. Your daily values may be higher or lower depending on your calorie needs.**

** Percent Daily Values listed below are intended for adults and children over 4 years of age. Foods represented or purported to be for use by infants, children less than 4 years of age, pregnant women, or lactating women shall use the RDI's that are specified for the intended group provided by the FDA.

| | Calories: | 2,000 | 2,500 |
|---|---|---|---|
| Total Fat | Less than | 65g | 80g |
| Sat. Fat | Less than | 20g | 25g |
| Cholesterol | Less than | 300mg | 300mg |
| Sodium | Less than | 2400mg | 2400mg |
| Potassium | | 3500mg | 3500mg |
| Total Carbohydrate | | 300mg | 375mg |
| Dietary Fiber | | 25mg | 30mg |

Calories per gram:

Fat 9    Carbohydrate 4    Protein 4

Rating: 3.5/10

## Welch's Fruit Punch Berries N Cherries Fat Free 80 Calorie Fruit Snacks Pouches, .9 oz, 22ct

Fruit Punch: Juice from Concentrates (Apple, Grape, Pear, Peach, And Pineapple), Corn Syrup, Sugar, Modified Corn Starch, Fruit Purees (Apple, Pineapple, Orange And Cherry), Gelatin, Citric Acid, Lactic Acid, Natural And Artificial Flavors, Ascorbic Acid (Vitamin C), Alpha Tocopherol Acetate (Vitamin E), Vitamin A Palmitate, Sodium Citrate, Coconut Oil, Carnauba Wax, And Red 40. Berries 'n Cherries: Juice from Concentrates (Apple, Grape, Pear, Peach, And Pineapple), Corn Syrup, Sugar, Modified Corn Starch, Fruit Purees (Strawberry, Raspberry, Blackberry, Blueberry, And Cherry), Gelatin, Citric Acid, Lactic Acid, Natural And Artificial Flavors, Ascorbic Acid (Vitamin C), Alpha Tocopherol Acetate (Vitamin E), Vitamin A Palmitate, Sodium Citrate, Coconut Oil, Carnauba Wax, Red 40, And Blue 1.

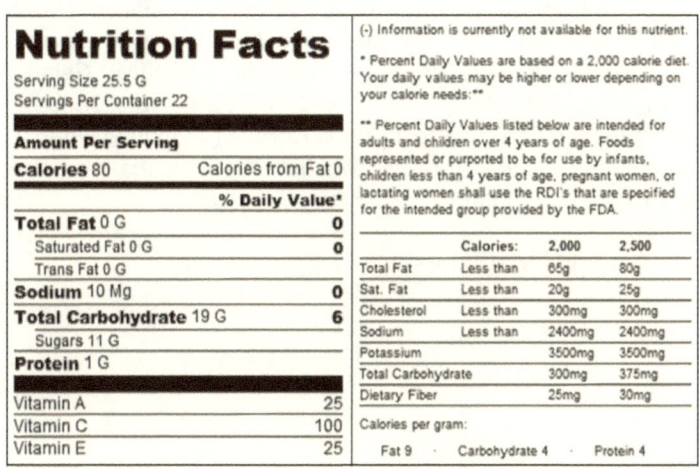

# Nutrition Facts

Serving Size 25.5 G
Servings Per Container 22

**Amount Per Serving**

| Calories 80 | Calories from Fat 0 |
|---|---|

| | % Daily Value* |
|---|---|
| **Total Fat** 0 G | 0 |
| Saturated Fat 0 G | 0 |
| Trans Fat 0 G | |
| **Sodium** 10 Mg | 0 |
| **Total Carbohydrate** 19 G | 6 |
| Sugars 11 G | |
| **Protein** 1 G | |

| | |
|---|---|
| Vitamin A | 25 |
| Vitamin C | 100 |
| Vitamin E | 25 |

(-) Information is currently not available for this nutrient.

* Percent Daily Values are based on a 2,000 calorie diet. Your daily values may be higher or lower depending on your calorie needs:**

** Percent Daily Values listed below are intended for adults and children over 4 years of age. Foods represented or purported to be for use by infants, children less than 4 years of age, pregnant women, or lactating women shall use the RDI's that are specified for the intended group provided by the FDA.

| | Calories: | 2,000 | 2,500 |
|---|---|---|---|
| Total Fat | Less than | 65g | 80g |
| Sat. Fat | Less than | 20g | 25g |
| Cholesterol | Less than | 300mg | 300mg |
| Sodium | Less than | 2400mg | 2400mg |
| Potassium | | 3500mg | 3500mg |
| Total Carbohydrate | | 300mg | 375mg |
| Dietary Fiber | | 25mg | 30mg |

Calories per gram:

Fat 9 · Carbohydrate 4 · Protein 4

High calorie, high carb, has 1 gram of protein
Rating: 5.5/10 Stars

# Welch's Island Fruits Fruit Snacks Pouches, 22 count

## Nutrition Facts

Serving Size 25.5 G
Servings Per Container 22

**Amount Per Serving**

**Calories** 80     Calories from Fat 0

| | % Daily Value* |
|---|---|
| **Total Fat** 0 G | 0 |
| Saturated Fat 0 G | 0 |
| Trans Fat 0 G | |
| **Sodium** 10 Mg | 0 |
| **Total Carbohydrate** 19 G | 6 |
| Sugars 11 G | |
| **Protein** 1 G | |
| Vitamin A | 25 |
| Vitamin C | 100 |
| Vitamin E | 25 |

(-) Information is currently not available for this nutrient.

* Percent Daily Values are based on a 2,000 calorie diet. Your daily values may be higher or lower depending on your calorie needs:**

** Percent Daily Values listed below are intended for adults and children over 4 years of age. Foods represented or purported to be for use by infants, children less than 4 years of age, pregnant women, or lactating women shall use the RDI's that are specified for the intended group provided by the FDA.

| | | Calories: | 2,000 | 2,500 |
|---|---|---|---|---|
| Total Fat | Less than | | 65g | 80g |
| Sat. Fat | Less than | | 20g | 25g |
| Cholesterol | Less than | | 300mg | 300mg |
| Sodium | Less than | | 2400mg | 2400mg |
| Potassium | | | 3500mg | 3500mg |
| Total Carbohydrate | | | 300mg | 375mg |
| Dietary Fiber | | | 25mg | 30mg |

Calories per gram:

Fat 9 · Carbohydrate 4 · Protein 4

Juice from Concentrates (Grape, Pear, Peach, Passion Fruit, And Pineapple), Corn Syrup, Sugar, Modified Corn Starch, Fruit Purees (Banana, Mango, Pineapple, And Kiwi), Gelatin, Citric Acid, Lactic Acid, Natural And Artificial Flavors, Ascorbic Acid (Vitamin C), Alpha Tocopheryl Acetate (Vitamin E), Vitamin A Palmitate, Sodium Citrate, Coconut Oil, Carnauba Wax, Red 4O, Yellow 5, And Blue 1.

Rating: 5.5/10 Stars

# Sunkist Mixed Fruit Fruit Flavored Snacks, 0.8 oz, 24 count

Fruit Juice Blend From Concentrate (Apple, Pear), Corn Syrup, Sugar, Modified Corn Starch. Contains 2% Or Less Of: Fruit Pectin, Vitamin C (Ascorbic Acid), Citric Acid, Dextrose, Sodium Citrate, Malic Acid, Potassium, Citrate, Mineral Oil, Natural Flavor, Carnauba Wax, Color (Red 40, Yellow 5, Blue 1), Beeswax.

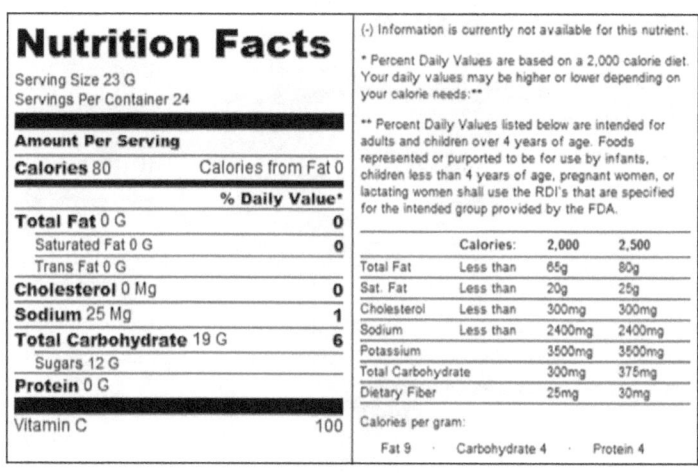

## Nutrition Facts

Serving Size 23 G
Servings Per Container 24

**Amount Per Serving**

**Calories** 80  Calories from Fat 0

|  | % Daily Value* |
|---|---|
| **Total Fat** 0 G | 0 |
| Saturated Fat 0 G | 0 |
| Trans Fat 0 G | |
| **Cholesterol** 0 Mg | 0 |
| **Sodium** 25 Mg | 1 |
| **Total Carbohydrate** 19 G | 6 |
| Sugars 12 G | |
| **Protein** 0 G | |
| Vitamin C | 100 |

(-) Information is currently not available for this nutrient.

* Percent Daily Values are based on a 2,000 calorie diet. Your daily values may be higher or lower depending on your calorie needs:**

** Percent Daily Values listed below are intended for adults and children over 4 years of age. Foods represented or purported to be for use by infants, children less than 4 years of age, pregnant women, or lactating women shall use the RDI's that are specified for the intended group provided by the FDA.

|  | | Calories: | 2,000 | 2,500 |
|---|---|---|---|---|
| Total Fat | Less than | | 65g | 80g |
| Sat. Fat | Less than | | 20g | 25g |
| Cholesterol | Less than | | 300mg | 300mg |
| Sodium | Less than | | 2400mg | 2400mg |
| Potassium | | | 3500mg | 3500mg |
| Total Carbohydrate | | | 300mg | 375mg |
| Dietary Fiber | | | 25mg | 30mg |

Calories per gram:
Fat 9 · Carbohydrate 4 · Protein 4

**Rating: 5.5/10 Stars**

# Mott's Medleys Assorted Fruit Fruit Flavored Snacks, 0.8 oz, 24 count

Less of: Fruit Pectin, Citric Fruit And Vegetable Juice Blend from Concentrate (Pear, Apple, Carrot), Corn Syrup, Sugar, Modified Corn Starch. Contains 2% Or Acid, Vitamin C (Ascorbic Acid), Dextrose, Sodium Citrate, Vegetable And Fruit Juice Added For Color, Malic Acid, Potassium Citrate, Mineral Oil+, Natural Flavor, Carnauba Wax, Beeswax. +Adds A Trivial Amount of Fat.

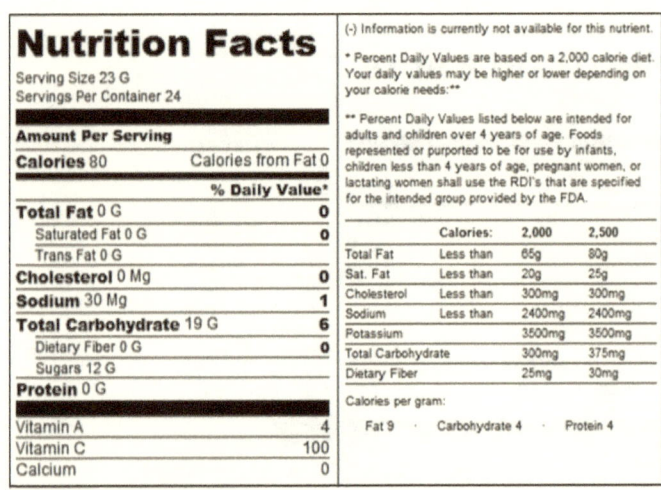

# Great Value Lemon/Grape/Strawberry/Orange Fruit Smiles Pouches, 42ct

Corn Syrup, Sugar, Fruit Juice Concentrate (Apple, Grape, Strawberry, Orange, Lemon), Modified Cornstarch, Cornstarch, Canola Oil, Contains Less Than 2% Of The Following: Malic Acid, Ascorbic Acid (Vitamin C), Natural And Artificial Flavors, Mineral Oil, Blue 1, Red 40, Yellow 5, Yellow 6, Carnauba Wax.

**Rating: 5.5 Stars**

# Kellogg's Disney/Pixar Finding Nemo Assorted Fruit Flavored Snacks, 20 CT

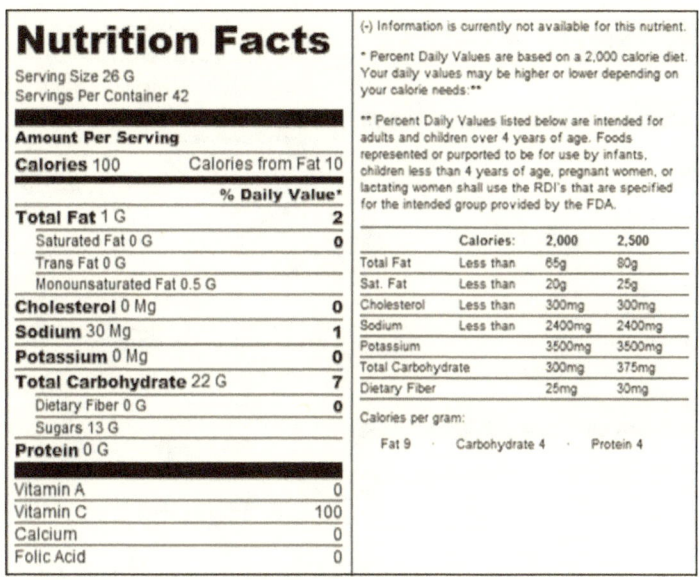

**Nutrition Facts**

Serving Size 26 G
Servings Per Container 42

**Amount Per Serving**

| Calories 100 | Calories from Fat 10 |
|---|---|

| | % Daily Value* |
|---|---|
| **Total Fat** 1 G | 2 |
| Saturated Fat 0 G | 0 |
| Trans Fat 0 G | |
| Monounsaturated Fat 0.5 G | |
| **Cholesterol** 0 Mg | 0 |
| **Sodium** 30 Mg | 1 |
| **Potassium** 0 Mg | 0 |
| **Total Carbohydrate** 22 G | 7 |
| Dietary Fiber 0 G | 0 |
| Sugars 13 G | |
| **Protein** 0 G | |

| Vitamin A | 0 |
|---|---|
| Vitamin C | 100 |
| Calcium | 0 |
| Folic Acid | 0 |

(-) Information is currently not available for this nutrient.

* Percent Daily Values are based on a 2,000 calorie diet. Your daily values may be higher or lower depending on your calorie needs:**

** Percent Daily Values listed below are intended for adults and children over 4 years of age. Foods represented or purported to be for use by infants, children less than 4 years of age, pregnant women, or lactating women shall use the RDI's that are specified for the intended group provided by the FDA.

| | | Calories: | 2,000 | 2,500 |
|---|---|---|---|---|
| Total Fat | Less than | | 65g | 80g |
| Sat. Fat | Less than | | 20g | 25g |
| Cholesterol | Less than | | 300mg | 300mg |
| Sodium | Less than | | 2400mg | 2400mg |
| Potassium | | | 3500mg | 3500mg |
| Total Carbohydrate | | | 300mg | 375mg |
| Dietary Fiber | | | 25mg | 30mg |

Calories per gram:

Fat 9 · Carbohydrate 4 · Protein 4

Corn Syrup, Sugar, Apple Puree Concentrate, Water, Modified Corn Starch, Gelatin, Contains Two Percent Or Less of Citric Acid, Ascorbic Acid (Vitamin C), Natural And Artificial Flavor, Coconut Oil*, Carnauba Wax, Red #40, Yellow #5, Sodium Citrate, Blue #1. *Adds A Trivial Amount of Fat.

**Rating: 5.5/10 Stars**

# Mott's Medleys Assorted Fruit Fruit Flavored Snacks, 0.8 oz, 24 count

## Nutrition Facts

Serving Size 23 G
Servings Per Container 24

**Amount Per Serving**

| **Calories** 80 | Calories from Fat 0 |
|---|---|

**% Daily Value\***

| | |
|---|---|
| **Total Fat** 0 G | 0 |
| Saturated Fat 0 G | 0 |
| Trans Fat 0 G | |
| **Cholesterol** 0 Mg | 0 |
| **Sodium** 30 Mg | 1 |
| **Total Carbohydrate** 19 G | 6 |
| Dietary Fiber 0 G | 0 |
| Sugars 12 G | |
| **Protein** 0 G | |
| Vitamin A | 4 |
| Vitamin C | 100 |
| Calcium | 0 |

(-) Information is currently not available for this nutrient.

\* Percent Daily Values are based on a 2,000 calorie diet. Your daily values may be higher or lower depending on your calorie needs:\*\*

\*\* Percent Daily Values listed below are intended for adults and children over 4 years of age. Foods represented or purported to be for use by infants, children less than 4 years of age, pregnant women, or lactating women shall use the RDI's that are specified for the intended group provided by the FDA.

| | Calories: | 2,000 | 2,500 |
|---|---|---|---|
| Total Fat | Less than | 65g | 80g |
| Sat. Fat | Less than | 20g | 25g |
| Cholesterol | Less than | 300mg | 300mg |
| Sodium | Less than | 2400mg | 2400mg |
| Potassium | | 3500mg | 3500mg |
| Total Carbohydrate | | 300mg | 375mg |
| Dietary Fiber | | 25mg | 30mg |

Calories per gram:

Fat 9 · Carbohydrate 4 · Protein 4

Fruit And Vegetable Juice Blend from Concentrate (Pear, Apple, Carrot), Corn Syrup, Sugar, Modified Corn Starch. Contains 2% Or Less of: Fruit Pectin, Citric Acid, Vitamin C (Ascorbic Acid), Dextrose, Sodium Citrate, Vegetable And Fruit Juice Added For Color, Malic Acid, Potassium Citrate, Mineral Oil+, Natural Flavor, Carnauba Wax, Beeswax. +Adds A Trivial Amount of Fat.

**Rating: 5.5 Stars**

# Fiber One Assorted Fruit Flavored Snacks

## Nutrition Facts

Serving Size 23 G
Servings Per Container 10

**Amount Per Serving**

| | |
|---|---|
| **Calories** 70 | Calories from Fat 0 |

**% Daily Value***

| | |
|---|---|
| **Total Fat** 0 G | **0** |
| Saturated Fat 0 G | **0** |
| Trans Fat 0 G | |
| **Cholesterol** 0 Mg | **0** |
| **Sodium** 25 Mg | **1** |
| **Total Carbohydrate** 19 G | **6** |
| Dietary Fiber 3 G | **10** |
| Sugars 10 G | |
| **Protein** 0 G | |
| Vitamin A | 0 |
| Vitamin C | 100 |
| Calcium | 0 |

(-) Information is currently not available for this nutrient.

* Percent Daily Values are based on a 2,000 calorie diet. Your daily values may be higher or lower depending on your calorie needs:**

** Percent Daily Values listed below are intended for adults and children over 4 years of age. Foods represented or purported to be for use by infants, children less than 4 years of age, pregnant women, or lactating women shall use the RDI's that are specified for the intended group provided by the FDA.

| | | Calories: | 2,000 | 2,500 |
|---|---|---|---|---|
| Total Fat | Less than | | 65g | 80g |
| Sat. Fat | Less than | | 20g | 25g |
| Cholesterol | Less than | | 300mg | 300mg |
| Sodium | Less than | | 2400mg | 2400mg |
| Potassium | | | 3500mg | 3500mg |
| Total Carbohydrate | | | 300mg | 375mg |
| Dietary Fiber | | | 25mg | 30mg |

Calories per gram:

Fat 9 · Carbohydrate 4 · Protein 4

Fruit Juice Blend from Concentrate (Pear, Apple), Sugar, Corn Syrup, Soluble Corn Fiber, Modified Corn Starch. Contains 2% Or Less of Fruit Pectin, Citric Acid, Vitamin C (Ascorbic Acid), Dextrose, Sodium Citrate, Malic Acid, Vegetable Juice And Fruit Juice Added For Color, Sunflower Oil+, Potassium Citrate, Natural Flavor, Carnauba Wax. +Adds A Trivial Amount of Fat.

**Rating: 6/10 Stars**

## Kellogg's Fruity Snacks Mixed Berry Assorted Fruit Flavored Snacks, 20 count

Ocean Spray Berrires & Cherries Fruit Flavoured Snacks, 0.8 OZ 24 count

Corn Syrup, Sugar, Apple Puree Concentrate, Water, Modified Corn Starch, Gelatin, Contains Two Percent Or Less of Citric Acid, Ascorbic Acid (Vitamin C), Natural And Artificial Flavor, Coconut Oil*, Carnauba Wax, Red #40, Yellow #5, Sodium Citrate, Blue #1. *Adds A Trivial Amount of Fat.

# Nutrition Facts

Serving Size 22 G
Servings Per Container 20

**Amount Per Serving**

**Calories** 70 — Calories from Fat 0

% Daily Value*

| | |
|---|---|
| **Total Fat** 0 G | 0 |
| Saturated Fat 0 G | 0 |
| Trans Fat 0 G | |
| **Cholesterol** 0 Mg | 0 |
| **Sodium** 0 Mg | 0 |
| **Total Carbohydrate** 17 G | 6 |
| Dietary Fiber 0 G | 0 |
| Sugars 11 G | |
| **Protein** <1 G | |

| | |
|---|---|
| Vitamin A | 0 |
| Vitamin C | 100 |
| Calcium | 0 |

(-) Information is currently not available for this nutrient.

* Percent Daily Values are based on a 2,000 calorie diet. Your daily values may be higher or lower depending on your calorie needs:**

** Percent Daily Values listed below are intended for adults and children over 4 years of age. Foods represented or purported to be for use by infants, children less than 4 years of age, pregnant women, or lactating women shall use the RDI's that are specified for the intended group provided by the FDA.

| | Calories: | 2,000 | 2,500 |
|---|---|---|---|
| Total Fat | Less than | 65g | 80g |
| Sat. Fat | Less than | 20g | 25g |
| Cholesterol | Less than | 300mg | 300mg |
| Sodium | Less than | 2400mg | 2400mg |
| Potassium | | 3500mg | 3500mg |
| Total Carbohydrate | | 300mg | 375mg |
| Dietary Fiber | | 25mg | 30mg |

Calories per gram:

Fat 9 · Carbohydrate 4 · Protein 4

# Ocean Spray Berries & Cherries Fruit Flavored Snacks, 0.8 oz, 24 count

Fruit Juice Blend from Concentrate (Pear, Apple, Cranberry), Corn Syrup, Sugar, Modified Corn Starch. Contains 2% Or Less of: Fruit Pectin, Citric Acid, Vitamin C (Ascorbic Acid), Dextrose, Sodium Citrate, Malic Acid, Vegetable Juice And Fruit Juice Added For Color, Sunflower Oil+, Potassium Citrate, Natural Flavor, Carnauba Wax. +Adds A Trivial Amount of Fat.

**Rating: 5.5/10 Stars**

## Winner: Fiber one assorted fruit flavoured snacks